SONOMA DIET 2025

110 Recipes The New Method to Lose Weight and Live Better A Journey Toward Health With the Diet of the Future

KLARLOCK

DISCLAIMER

This book aims to provide useful and informative material on the topics covered in the publication. It is sold with the understanding that the author and publisher are not engaged in rendering any personal medical, health care, or other professional services in the book. The reader should consult his or her physician, health care provider, or other competent professional before adopting any suggestions in this book or drawing any conclusions. The author and publisher expressly disclaim any responsibility for any liability, loss, or risk, personal or otherwise, arising, directly or indirectly, from the use and application of any contents of this book.

NOTE

All the recipes in this book are designed for four people. For this quantity, the ingredients indicated in the recipes must be considered. If you need to change the portion, it is recommended to proportionally adjust the doses of the ingredients. It is also recommended to carefully follow the preparation and cooking instructions to obtain the best result. In the context of this book, when we refer to "a cup" as a unit of measurement for ingredients, we mean using a standard kitchen cup with a capacity of approximately 240 milliliters. It is essential to use a measuring cup to get the right quantities of ingredients. If you don't have a measuring cup, you can use a graduated measuring cup, making sure to correctly correspond to the proportions indicated. Here are some examples 1 Cup of flour 100 gr. 1 cup of rice 200 gr. 1 Cup of Quinoa 200 gr

TABLE OF CONTENT

INTRODUCTION TO THE SONOMA DIET 5

ORIGIN OF THE SONOMA DIET

WHAT IS THE SONOMA DIET

STRUCTURE AND PHASES OF THE SONOMA DIET

BENEFITS OF THE SONOMA DIET

RECIPES APPETIZERS

29 LENTIL MEATBALLS

32 BEET HUMMUS

34 COD CARPACCIO

37 COURGETTE FLOWERS STUFFED WITH RICE, BREADED AND FRIED

40 SPRING ROLLS WITH CRAB MEAT, VEGETABLES AND SOY

43 SMOKED SALMON WITH SWEDISH DILL

45 SEAFOOD PIZZAS WITH CLAMS AND TOMATO

48 TORTILLAS WITH PAPAYA AND SPICY SUMMER VEGETABLES: FROM THE CARIBBEAN

51 SUMMER STUFFED PEPPERS

RECIPES FIRST DISHES

55 COLD PASTA WITH CREAM OF TUNA AND TOMATOES

57 PASTA WITH BOTTARGA WITH FRESH TOMATO

60 LINGUINE WITH WALNUT PESTO, PINE NUTS AND MINT

62 CREAM OF PEAS AND SPRING ONIONS

65 LIGHT SPINACH CREAM

68 THAI-STYLE SHRIMP, MUSHROOM AND ASPARAGUS SOUP

71 ROASTED TOMATO CREAM

74 VEGETARIAN AND DIETARY COZY SOUP

77 FRENCH ONION SOUP

80 SPAGHETTI WITH RANCETTO

83 CUCUMBER SPAGHETTI WITH TOMATOES, BASIL AND OLIVES

85 TAGLIATELLE WITH BROCCOLETTI AND WALNUT CREAM WITH POCHÈ EGGS

88 BUCKWHEAT WITH VEGETABLES AND CHESTNUTS WITH RED CABBAGE CREAM

91 MALTAGLIATI WITH LEEKS AND MUSHROOM AND HAZELNUT SAUCE

94 PISTACHIO GNOCCHI IN PUMPKIN SAUCE

96 CHESTNUT TAGLIOLINI WITH LEEKS IN RED WINE AND ALMONDS

99 EGG TAGLIOLINI WITH LENTIL RAGU AND PORCINI MUSHROOMS

102 BREAD PIZZAS WITH LEEKS, BRIE AND HAZELNUTS

105 SAFFRON TAGLIOLINI IN FRESH LEEK AND PORCINI CREAM

108 PINK RICOTTA AND BEETROOT GNOCCHI WITH SAGE

110 BARLEY AND BORLOTTI BEAN SALAD IN YOGURT SAUCE

112 BUTTERFLIES WITH THYME SCENTED PEPPERS

114 SPAGHETTI WITH GREEN BEANS, BASIL AND CHILI PEPPER

116 SMALL WARM TIMBALES WITH AUBERGINES AND OLIVES

119 SPELLED PENNETTE WITH PARMESAN AND RATATUJA

122 SPAGHETTI WITH DOUBLE TOMATO WITH BASIL

125 POTATO GNOCCHI WITH PEAS AND BASIL VEGETABLES

128 ASPARAGUS LASAGNA

131 MEDITERRANEAN OVEN STUFFED ARTICHOKES

134 GREEN LINGUINE WITH SPINACH AND GOAT'S RICOTTA

136 TURNIP SPATZLE WITH PINE NUTS

138 WHITE ARTICHOKE AND WALNUT LASAGNA

140 WHOLE BAVETTE WITH ARTICHOKES IN CURRY ONION SAUCE

142 PIZZOCCHERI WITH TOPINAMBUR AND CHICORY

144 TORTIGLIONE CARBONARA

147 CREAMY ORECCHIETTE WITH PORCINI MUSHROOMS AND PARSLEY

149 ROMAN-STYLE GNOCCHI WITH WHITE POLENTA WITH WALNUTS AND SAGE

152 BAKED WHOLE WHOLE PASTA WITH PEPPERS AND PECORINO

154 ANDALUSIAN GAZPACHO

157 CHICKPEA, FONTINA AND DRIED TOMATOES CAKE

159 WHOLE WHEAT PENS WITH SPRING ONIONS AND GREEK YOGURT

161 BULGUR SALAD WITH PEAS, TOMATOES, BASIL

164 CREAM OF BLACK CHICKPEAS WITH BEANS, CARROTS AND POTATOES

166 BUCATINI ARRIVAL WITH SAFFRON GREEN BEANS

169 CARROT GNOCCHI IN FRESH BEAN BEAN CREAM

RECIPES SECOND DISHES

173 PAN-FISHED SWORDFISH

175 GRILLED SALMON FILLET

178 MEATBALLS WITH PESTO

180 BAKED RABBIT

182 TYROLEAN GROSTL

184 BAKED HAKE FILLETS

186 OVEN STUFFED POTATOES WITH CHEESE AND HAM

188 CAVAGE MEATBALLS

190 BAKED DUCK

192 BAKED SALMON GRATIN

194 VEGETABLE CRUMBLE

197 TUNA MEATBALLS

199 BAKED HAKE WITH TOMATOES AND OLIVES

201 CHICKEN WITH LEMON

203 BAKED PRAWNS

205 VEAL STRIPS WITH ARTICHOKES

207 MEATLOAF WITH ARTICHOKES

210 TURKEY ROLL STUFFED WITH COURGETTES AND HAM

212 TUNA FILLET IN PISTACHIO CRUST

214 SPINACH OMELETTE WITHOUT EGGS

216 GUINEA-STYLE CACCIATORA WITH OLIVES

218 CUTTLEFISH AND ARTICHOKES

221 CAULIFLOWER BURGER

223 STUFFED ARTICHOKES WITHOUT MEAT

226 CARROT PANCAKES

229 CHICKEN SKEWERS WITH SOY

231 AUBERGINE AND LENTIL MEATBALLS

233 CAULIFLOWER CUTLETS

235 OMELETTE WITH FAVE BEANS, PEAS AND GREEN BEANS

238 LENTIL BURGER

240 MEXICAN VEGETARIAN ENCHILADAS WITH BEANS AND VEGETABLES

243 PEPPER AND ZUCCHINI OMELETTE

245 POTATO AND HAM PIE

247 COD WITH PEARS

250 SEAFOOD SALAD WITH MUSSELS AND CELERY

253 PORK FILLET WITH PEACHES

255 AUBERGINES STUFFED WITH TUNA

258 PEPPERS STUFFED WITH QUINOA AND VEGETABLES

261 CHICKEN WITH PEPPERS

264 STURGEON TURKEY WITH VEGETABLES

266 CHICKEN ROLLS WITH PESTO

268 SAVORY PIE WITH GREEN BEANS AND COURGETTES

271 SALAD OF MOSCARDINI AND GREEN BEANS

274 CHICKEN IN SWEET AND SOUR SAUCE

277 THAI CHICKEN BITES WITH CURRY AND COCONUT MILK

279 OMELETTE WITH AGRETTI

SIDE DISH RECIPES

282 SPINACH AND STRAWBERRY SALAD

284 STEAMED BROCCOLI WITH ALMONDS

286 QUINOA WITH GRILLED VEGETABLES

288 ROASTED ASPARAGUS WITH PARMESAN

290 TOMATO AND CUCUMBER SALAD

292 ROASTED CARROTS WITH HONEY AND THYME

294 BAKED CAULIFLOWER WITH TURMERIC AND CUMIN

296 SPELLED SALAD WITH VEGETABLES

298 PEPPERS STUFFED WITH COUSCOUS

301 GRILLED MARINATED COURGETTES

INTRODUCTION TO THE SONOMA DIET

The Sonoma Diet is a diet that draws inspiration from Mediterranean cuisine, known for promoting a healthy and balanced lifestyle. This diet takes its name from the Sonoma Valley region of California, famous for its vineyards and cuisine. Basic Principles of the Sonoma Diet 1. Focus on Whole Foods: The diet focuses on unprocessed, whole foods, such as fruits, vegetables, whole grains, lean proteins and healthy fats. 2. Portion Control: More than counting calories, the Sonoma Diet emphasizes portion control, promoting the idea of eating mindfully. 3. Plate Divided into Sectors: The plate is divided into three main sectors: half of the plate is reserved for fruit and vegetables, a quarter for lean proteins and the last quarter for whole grains. 4. Key Foods: Some foods are given special consideration beneficial and are encouraged, such as nuts, olive oil, tomatoes, berries, grapes, spinach and salmon. 5. Three Phases: The diet is divided into three phases: Wave 1 (First Wave): Duration of 10 days, aimed at eliminating cravings for sugars and refined carbohydrates. Wave 2 (Second Wave): Main phase where you develop healthy eating habits and continue to lose weight. Wave 3 (Third Wave): Long-term maintenance phase to stabilize the weight achieved. Benefits of the Sonoma Diet Sustainable Weight Loss: With an emphasis on whole foods and controlled portions, the diet promotes gradual, sustainable weight loss. Cardiovascular Health: The diet, rich in healthy fats and low in saturated fats, is beneficial for heart health. Reduced Risk of Chronic Diseases: Key foods promoted in the diet are known to reduce the risk of chronic diseases such as type 2 diabetes and some forms of cancer.

Breakfast Menu Example: Greek yogurt with fresh berries and a spoonful of chia seeds. Lunch: Mixed salad with spinach, tomatoes, avocado, walnuts and grilled chicken breast, dressed with olive oil and balsamic vinegar. Dinner: Baked salmon with a portion of quinoa and grilled vegetables. Snack: Fresh fruit, a handful of almonds or a portion of hummus with carrots and celery. Final Thoughts The Sonoma Diet promotes a healthy, sustainable lifestyle, rather than a quick fix for weight loss. Its emphasis on fresh, whole foods, paired with portion control and a mindful approach to food, makes it an attractive choice for those looking to improve their overall health and well-being.

ORIGIN OF THE SONOMA DIET

The Sonoma Diet draws inspiration from Mediterranean cuisine and lifestyle, known for their health and longevity benefits. Origins of the Sonoma Diet 1. The Sonoma Region: Located in California, Sonoma Valley is famous for its vineyards, wine production and gourmet cuisine. The region is often compared to wine-growing areas of the Mediterranean, such as Tuscany in Italy and Provence in France. This similarity inspired them to develop a diet that reflected Sonoma's culinary culture and laid-back lifestyle. 2. Mediterranean Cuisine: The diet is based on the principles of Mediterranean cuisine, which includes an abundance of fresh fruits and vegetables, whole grains, legumes, nuts, olive oil and fish. Scientific studies have shown that the Mediterranean diet can reduce the risk of cardiovascular disease, improve metabolic health and promote longevity. 3. Influence of Blue Zones:

"Blue Zones" are regions of the world where people live longer and healthier lives. These areas share similar dietary habits, including a diet high in unprocessed foods, low consumption of red meat and dairy products, and high intake of legumes and fish. The Sonoma Diet incorporates many of these principles to promote a long, healthy life. Inspiring Principles 1. Whole, Unprocessed Foods: The diet places a strong emphasis on fresh, unprocessed foods, similar to those consumed in traditional Mediterranean and Blue Zones diets. 2. Eating Awareness: Eating mindfully and enjoying every bite is another key principle of the Sonoma Diet. This approach promotes a healthy relationship with food and helps avoid overeating. 3. Balance and Moderation: The Sonoma Diet is not restrictive; rather, it encourages balance and moderation. There are no completely forbidden foods, but it is important to eat in moderation and choose appropriate portions.

4. Enjoyment of Food: One of the distinctive aspects of the Sonoma Diet is the emphasis on enjoyment of food. The diet encourages you to enjoy meals, using fresh and tasty ingredients, and to consider meals as a moment of pleasure and conviviality. Conclusion The Sonoma Diet is an eating plan that combines the best of Mediterranean cuisine with the relaxed lifestyle of the Sonoma Valley. Through an emphasis on whole foods, portion control and dietary awareness, the diet promotes optimal health and overall well-being, making it an attractive choice for those looking to improve their dietary lifestyle.

WHAT IS THE SONOMA DIET

The Sonoma Diet is a dietary program inspired by the Mediterranean cuisine and culture of California's Sonoma Valley. the diet focuses on fresh, whole and nutritious foods, promoting a healthy and balanced lifestyle. Here are the fundamental principles of the Sonoma Diet: Fundamental Principles 1. Focus on Whole Foods: The diet is based on fruits, vegetables, whole grains, lean proteins and healthy fats, minimizing processed and refined foods. 2. Portion Control: Instead of counting calories, the Sonoma Diet emphasizes portion control. The plate is divided into sections: half for fruits and vegetables, a quarter for lean proteins and the last quarter for whole grains. 3. Key Foods: Certain foods, such as nuts, olive oil, tomatoes, berries, grapes, spinach and salmon, are especially encouraged for their nutritional benefits. Structure of the Diet The Sonoma Diet is structured into three main phases, called

"Wave" (waves): 1. Wave 1 (First Wave): This phase lasts 10 days and is intended to eliminate cravings for sugars and refined carbohydrates, establishing the foundation for a healthy diet. 2. Wave 2 (Second Wave): The main phase of the diet, during which you continue to develop healthy eating habits and lose weight sustainably. During this phase, certain foods such as whole grains and more varieties of fruit are gradually reintroduced. 3. Wave 3 (Third Wave): The long-term maintenance phase, which lasts indefinitely. In this phase, you continue to follow the principles of the diet with greater flexibility, maintaining the weight you have achieved and a healthy lifestyle. Benefits of the Sonoma Diet Sustainable Weight Loss: Thanks to its emphasis on whole foods and portion control, the diet promotes gradual, sustainable weight loss. Cardiovascular Health: Rich in healthy fats and low in saturated fats, the diet is beneficial for heart health. Pleasure of Food:

STRUCTURE AND PHASES OF THE SONOMA DIET

The Sonoma Diet is structured into three main phases, called "Waves", which progressively guide participants towards healthier eating habits and long-term maintenance of body weight. Here is a detailed description of each phase: Wave 1: First Wave Duration: 10 days Objective: This phase is designed to eliminate cravings for sugars and refined carbohydrates, helping you break bad eating habits and kickstart weight loss. Features: Elimination of Specific Foods: During Wave 1, refined sugars, refined grains, sweets, alcohol, and highly processed foods are excluded. Focus on Healthy Foods: The diet focuses on lean proteins, non-starchy vegetables, limited fruit, healthy fats and low-fat dairy products. Controlled Portions: Portions are carefully controlled to promote calorie reduction without the need to count calories. Sample Menu: Breakfast: Scrambled eggs with spinach and tomatoes. Lunch: Chicken salad with mixed vegetables and olive oil. Dinner: Grilled fish fillet with steamed broccoli. Snack: Celery sticks with hummus. Wave 2: Second Wave Duration: Until you reach your desired weight Objective: The main phase of the diet, where you develop healthy eating habits and continue to lose weight sustainably. Features: Reintroduction of Foods: Some foods such as whole grains, more varieties of fruit and red wine in moderate quantities are gradually reintroduced. Balanced Diet: Emphasizes a balance of proteins, carbohydrates and healthy fats. Variety and Moderation: A wider range of foods is permitted, but always with attention to portions and food quality. Sample Menu: Breakfast: Greek yogurt with fresh strawberries and nuts. Lunch: Turkey wrap with lettuce, tomatoes, avocado and a wholemeal tortilla. Dinner: Chicken breast grill with quinoa and roasted vegetables. Snack: Apple with almond butter. Wave 3: Third Wave Duration: Indefinite, for long-term maintenance Objective: Maintain the weight achieved and continue to follow a healthy lifestyle. Features: Sustainability: The diet is designed to be sustainable in the long term, without rigid restrictions. Flexibility: Allows greater flexibility in food choices, while still promoting healthy foods and moderate portions. Lifestyle: Encourages a lifestyle approach, rather than a temporary diet, incorporating principles of mindful eating and regular physical activity. Conclusion The wave structure of the Sonoma Diet allows a gradual approach to weight loss and improving eating habits, promoting a sustainable transition towards a healthy and balanced diet. Each phase is designed to promote well-being and help participants maintain long-term results.

BENEFITS OF THE SONOMA DIET

The Sonoma Diet offers numerous health and wellness benefits, thanks to its balanced approach and focus on fresh, whole foods. Here are some of the main benefits: 1. Gradual and Sustainable Weight Loss: The Sonoma Diet promotes gradual weight loss through portion control and the elimination of refined foods and sugars, avoiding the drastic calorie restrictions of yoyo diets. Weight Maintenance: The three phases of the diet help establish long-term healthy eating habits, making it easier to maintain the weight achieved. 2. Cardiovascular Health Healthy Fats: Inclusion of healthy fats such as olive oil, nuts and omega3-rich fish helps reduce the risk of cardiovascular disease. Cholesterol Reduction: A diet rich in fruits, vegetables and whole grains helps keep cholesterol levels low bad cholesterol (LDL) and improve good cholesterol (HDL) levels. 3. Blood Sugar Control Low Glycemic Index Carbohydrates: Emphasis on whole grains and reduction of refined sugars helps stabilize blood sugar levels: The diet reduces blood sugar fluctuations that cause sudden cravings and excessive hunger. 4. Improved Digestion Rich in Fibre: The high presence of fruit, vegetables and whole grains promotes good digestion and prevents problems such as constipation. Hydration: The diet encourages adequate water intake, which is important for healthy digestion. 5. General Wellbeing Nutrient Richness: The variety of fresh, whole foods provides a wide range of vitamins, minerals and antioxidants essential for optimal functioning of the body. Increased Energy: A balanced diet contributes to more stable and improved energy levels, reducing the feeling of tiredness. 6. Mental Health Conscious Eating:

The diet promotes a mindful approach to eating, helping you develop a healthy relationship with food and reduce food-related stress. Enjoyment of Food: By encouraging you to enjoy meals and treat food as a pleasure, the Sonoma Diet can improve emotional well-being and quality of life. 7. Reduce the Risk of Chronic Diseases Antioxidants and Phytonutrients: Key foods in the diet, such as berries, tomatoes and leafy greens, are rich in antioxidants that protect cells from damage and reduce the risk of cancer and other chronic diseases. Reduced Inflammation: Anti-inflammatory foods included in the diet, such as salmon and walnuts, help reduce systemic inflammation, associated with many chronic diseases. 8. Longevity Blue Zones Principles: The Sonoma Diet incorporates eating habits observed in "Blue Zones," areas of the world where people live longer and healthier lives, promoting long, healthy lives.

RECIPES
APPETIZERS

LENTIL MEATBALLS

Execution: easy

Preparation time: 15 minutes

+10 minutes of cooking

+ 30 minutes of rest in the refrigerator

Low price

Ingredients for 4 people:

500 g of already cooked lentils

1 fresh egg

1 potato

2 slices of canned bread

2 tablespoons grated parmesan

milk to taste breadcrumbs to taste

parsley to taste

seed oil to taste salt and pepper to taste

Preparation

Wash the potato well and cook it with its skin in boiling salted water until it becomes soft. In the meantime, remove the crust from the bread slices and let the crumbs soak in the milk. Once the potato has been boiled, peel it, cut it into small pieces and place it in a large bowl. Add the already cooked lentils, work the two ingredients with the tines of a fork and, when you have obtained a rather consistent but homogeneous puree with them, add the shelled egg and the crushed breadcrumbs. Knead the dough with your hands for 23 minutes; Also add the chopped parsley, 2 tablespoons of breadcrumbs and the grated parmesan. I season everything with a pinch of salt and so on pinch of pepper and continue to work until you obtain a uniform mixture. Then divide it into 16 small piles and fan out as many meatballs of the same size; Place them on a tray covered with kitchen paper and let them harden in the refrigerator for 30 minutes. After this time, Tioral comes out of the refrigerator and passes each one in breadcrumbs, being careful not to leave them uncovered. Pour plenty of seed oil into a large pan and, as soon as it has become hot but not yet to the point of smoking, add the meatballs and fry them until they have taken on a nice golden color over their entire surface. Then drain them, using a slotted spoon so that the oil drips off, place them on a sheet of absorbent paper and gently pat them dry with another sheet to remove excess grease. Finally,

BEET HUMMUS

Execution: easy

Time needed: 10 minutes

Low price

Ingredients for 4 people:

300 g of pre-cooked red beetroot

300 g of pre-cooked chickpeas

1 lemon

60 g of tahini sauce

1/2 clove of garlic

1 teaspoon paprika powder

1 scant teaspoon of cumin powder

6070 g of olive or sesame oil

raw carrots to decorate as desired

salt to taste

Preparation

Drain the chickpeas from their conservation water, rinse them and drain them; Cut the pre-cooked beetroot into chunks. Place the two ingredients in the blender glass, add the filtered lemon juice, 1/2 clove of garlic in skin, papal and cumin powder, and a pinch of salt. Turn on the mixer and blend everything intermittently, adding the oil little by little and possibly diluting the mixture with a little water only if necessary, softening it until you obtain a full-bodied and uniform cream. Prepare it in a bowl, decorate it, if you want, with fresh chopped mixture or with toasted sesame seeds or slices of raw carrot, as I do to create a pleasant color contrast, and serve it on the table.

COD CARPACCIO

Execution: easy

Time needed: 10 minutes

+ 4 hours of marinade

Low price

Ingredients for 4 people:

Already a cod fillet

Desolate and dejected by 700 g

2 cloves of garlic

2 lemons

peppercorns to taste

extra virgin olive oil to taste

Salt and pepper to taste

Preparation

Wash the cod fillet, dry it carefully with kitchen paper, remove the skin and place it on the cutting board. Remove any thorns remaining in the pulp, cut them into thin slices diagonally (as is done when manually slicing raw ham) with the help of a very sharp knife, then arrange them in a single layer in a large flat pan. Squeeze the lemons and pour the juice into a bowl, add a pinch of salt, a few grains of crushed pepper, the cloves and pieces of peeled garlic, and 2 glasses of extra virgin olive oil, emulsify everything with the tines of a fork and irritate the cod slices with the marinade obtained. Cover the baking dish with cling film, transfer it to the refrigerator and leave the too-cold cod to marinate for 45 hours, ringing the slices 1 or 2 times. After this time, drain the cod carpaccio, place it on the serving plate, season it with a drizzle of oil, freshly ground pepper and, if you want, with lemon juice or balsamic vinegar, and serve on the table accompanied with a vegetable salad to taste or with a mix of citrus fruits and raw vegetables.

COURGETTE FLOWERS STUFFED WITH BREADED AND FRIED RICE

Execution: easy

Time: 15 minutes

+20 minutes of cooking

Low price

Ingredients for 4 people:

12 courgette flowers (or squash)

100 grams of rice

150 g of courgettes, 1 onion

30 g of grated parmesan

1 large egg or 2 small ones

breadcrumbs to taste

extra virgin olive oil to taste

peanut oil for frying to taste

Salt and pepper to taste

Preparation

Clean the courgettes by removing the ends, rinse them, dry them well, cut them into julienne strips and set aside. Peel the onion, wash it, dry it, chop it, transfer it to a large pan and brown it briefly in extra virgin olive oil. When the mixture has become transparent, add the rice and toast it, stirring with a wooden spoon. Add the courgettes and cook them for about 2 minutes over a low heat. Then pour in the hot water a little at a time, waiting for it to be absorbed by the rice before adding the rest. Cook over low heat for 1015 minutes and, once the rice has reached al dente and dried, remove the pan from the heat, add

The grated parmesan, salt and pepper mix everything together delicately and leave to cool. In the meantime, remove the bitter pistil, the lateral growths and the stem of the courgette flower, being careful not to break them; Rinse and dry them very carefully. Then widen them, stuff them in the center with the now cold rice, close them well and dip them first in the beaten egg and then in the breadcrumbs. Fry them in abundant boiling peanut oil for 34 minutes and, when they have become golden, drain them with a slotted spoon, and gently pat them dry with kitchen paper to remove excess grease. Then serve your appetizing and crunchy courgette flowers stuffed with rice and fried so that they can be consumed piping hot.

SPRING ROLLS WITH CRAB MEAT, VEGETABLES AND SOY

Ingredients for 4 people:

12 large sheets of pasta

Give him frozen spring rolls

300 grams of crab meat

in the natural box, 1 fresh egg

80 grams of soy vermicelli

1 onion, 1 clove of garlic, 1 carrot

250 grams of red cabbage

3 tablespoons of extra virgin olive oil

50 grams of corn starch

1 tablespoon soy sauce

peanut oil for frying to taste

Salt and pepper to taste

Preparation

Remove the sheets of phyllo pastry you will
need from the freezer and let them thaw; Soak
the Shiitake mushrooms in water that drops to
40° for 1 hour to make them soft and then
drain them well and cut them into thin slices.
Clean the vegetables, wash them and dry them
well; Cut the carrot into julienne strips, thinly
slice the red cabbage, remove the skin from
the onion and garlic and chop them. Put a pan
with some water on the heat and, when it
starts to boil, add the whole skein of soya
spaghetti without destroying it, add the salt,
turn off the heat, cover with the lid, leave
them in the boiling water for about 2 minutes;
Then drain them, pass them under cold water
and keep them aside. Heat 2 tablespoons of
extra virgin olive oil in the wok, and add the
crab au naturel

the pulp and the chopped onion and garlic; Season with salt and pepper and brown briefly for about 1 minute before turning off the heat. Add the bowl of cooked vermicelli, pre-prepared vegetables, mushrooms, remaining oil and soy sauce and mix well. Open the sheets of spring roll pastry on the work surface, fill them with a little of the vegetable and vermicelli mixture, distribute the crab meat on top, fold 2 parallel sides and roll the sheets along the folded sides and close with the egg white egg. Brush the surface of the rolls obtained with the beaten egg, dip them in the cornstarch, shake them well to remove the excess, and fry them in plenty of boiling seed oil. Then drain them on kitchen paper and cut each roll into 23 pieces before serving them hot

SMOKED SALMON WITH SWEDISH DILL

Ingredients for 4 people:

400 grams of salmon smoked slices

1 sprig of fresh dill

2 cucumbers

4 tablespoons of mustard

2 tablespoons of apple cider vinegar

2 teaspoons dry white wine

8 tablespoons of extra virgin olive oil

4 slices of rye bread

Salt and pepper to taste

Preparation

of smoked salmon with Swedish dill sauce
Wash the fresh dill, dry it very well and chop
it, keeping 2 stalks aside. Prepare the Aneth
sauce as used in Nordic countries: emulsify
the chopped aromatic herb, apple cider
vinegar and dry white wine, mustard and
extra virgin olive oil in a bowl and then season
with salt and pepper. Rinse the cucumber, dry
it well, cut it into rather thin slices, place it in
a colander over the sink and let it rest for
about 20 minutes, the time needed to spread
the vegetable water. Arrange the slices of
smoked fish on 4 individual plates and
decorate them with the drained cucumber
slices, the coarsely chopped dandy stems kept
on one side and the rye bread cut into
triangles. Finally, salmon with Swedish dill
sauce is interconnected and served to the
table.

SEAFOOD PIZZAS WITH CLAMS AND TOMATO

Difficulty: medium

Preparation: about 25 minutes

Ingredients for 4 people:

800 grams of pizza bread dough

1 kilo of clams

3032 tablespoons of tomato puree

1 glass of dry white wine

6 tablespoons of extra virgin olive oil

2 bay leaves

6 sprigs of fresh thyme

salt to taste pepper to taste

Preparation

Drain the clams in fresh water with a handful of coarse salt for 23 hours in the refrigerator; then drain them, rinse them and place them in a large pot. Add 2 tablespoons of EVO oil, 4 sprigs of thyme (previously washed and dried), the bay leaves, a grind of pepper and let them open over high heat. While the shell valves begin to open, pour the glass of white wine over it and let most of the alcohol content evaporate. When the clams have opened: drain them, keep the cooking water aside and let them cool. Take the ready bread dough, place it on the cutting board and divide it into 18 loaves: roll out 16 of them on the work surface with the help of a rolling pin, giving each one a flat, oval shape. Arrange the pizzas obtained on the baking tray covered with baking paper and then roll out the 2 remaining loaves, cut 32 strips and arrange them on the edges of the pizzas, giving them the shape of a wave.

Preheat the oven to maximum temperature. Spread 2 tablespoons of tomato puree on each pizza, season it with a pinch of salt and a (little) drizzle of extra virgin olive oil and, when the oven is hot, insert the plate inside, close the door tightly and cook the pizzas for approximately 810 minutes. In the meantime, remove the shells from the molluscs, leaving some whole for decoration, and, when the pizzas are ready and out of the oven, distribute the seafood evenly on their surface. Filter approximately 2 tablespoons of the clam cooking water through a sieve, add them to the remaining oil and the remaining chopped fresh thyme leaves, mix carefully with a wooden spoon and pour the resulting sauce onto the pizzas. Cook the marinated pizzas with clams in a preheated oven at 220° for about 1 minute and,

TORTILLAS WITH PAPAYA AND SPICY SUMMER VEGETABLES: FROM THE CARIBBEAN

Execution: easy

Preparation: 20 minutes

+ 1/2 hour of rest

Ingredients for 6 people:

1/2 ripe papaya

2 firm, ripe tomatoes

1/2 yellow pepper

1/2 green pepper

1 white onion, 2 limes

2 packs of ready-made tortillas

1 pepper, salt to taste b

3 sprigs of fresh mint

Preparation

Rinse the tomatoes, cut the skin with a cross cut, blanch them for about thirty seconds in boiling water, immerse them briefly in cold water, remove the skin, seeds and core; then cut them into cubes, season them with salt and set them aside. Peel the onion, clean it, chop it finely, season with salt and sprinkle it with the squeezed and filtered juice of 1 lime. Remove the external peel from the papaya, remove the internal seeds and cut it into cubes; also cut the peppers into cubes after cleaning them, removing the core, seeds and white skin. Wash the mint, dry it (damp it carefully with kitchen paper), break it into pieces lift it with your hands and chop the chilli very finely. Place all the ingredients in a large bowl, sprinkle them with the juice of the other lime passed through a sieve, salt everything and mix delicately with a wooden spoon. Transfer the bowl to the refrigerator, cover it with cling film and let the papaya and spicy vegetable mixture rest for about 30 minutes before serving it, accompanied by the tortillas, on individual plates.

SUMMER STUFFED PEPPERS

Execution: easy

Preparation: about 30 minutes

Ingredients for 6 people:

6 fresh, hard peppers;

6 salted anchovies;

1 tablespoon of salted capers;

1 handful of pitted black olives;

3 eggs;

34 not too ripe tomatoes;

23 potatoes

extra virgin olive oil to taste;

fine salt and white pepper to taste

Preparation

of mum's summer stuffed peppers. Wash the
tomatoes, dry them and cut them into fillets or
small pieces. Boil the potatoes in their skins,
then remove the skins and cut them into
cubes. Cook the eggs in a saucepan containing
boiling water until they become hard-boiled;
then pass them under cold running water,
remove the shell and cut them into cubes.
Clean the salted anchovies, cut them into
fillets, pass them under running water and cut
them into small pieces. Rinse the capers under
cold running water to remove the salt, squeeze
them gently, dry them and set them aside in a
small bowl.

Wash the peppers, dry them and place them in the oven to cook until the outer film is golden (this step is used to easily remove the skin from the peppers and make them look like "sachets". Then remove the core, the seeds inside, and the burnt peel, wash and dry them carefully, also dabbing the inside with kitchen paper. Place all the other ingredients in a large bowl, add a few tablespoons of extra virgin olive oil, add salt, season with white pepper, mix gently with a wooden spoon and leave to rest for 5 minutes, fill the peppers with the mixture, place them on a serving plate, garnish with chopped parsley and serve this tasty summer dish at room temperature or slightly cold.

RECIPES
FIRST DISHES

COLD PASTA WITH CREAM OF TUNA AND TOMATOES

Execution: easy

Time: 10 minutes +

20 minutes of cooling

Low price

Ingredients for 4 people:

360 g of short pasta

250 g of tuna in oil

23 tomatoes, 1/2 lemon

5 tablespoons of mayonnaise

extra virgin olive oil to taste

Salt and pepper to taste

Preparation

Pour plenty of cold water into a large saucepan, heat it and, as soon as it starts bring to the boil, add the salt, add the pasta, mix and boil for 1 minute less than the time indicated on the package. While the pasta is cooking, wash the tomatoes, drain them, dry them, cut them first into slices and then into cubes, put them in a bowl, season them with a drizzle of extra virgin olive oil, salt, pepper and, if you like, even a little ' of fresh or dried garlic. After draining the tuna well, transfer it to the glass of the food processor, add the mayonnaise and the filtered juice of 1/2 lemon and blend everything until you obtain a smooth cream. When the pasta is cooked al dente, drain it, pass it quickly under the jet of water to stop cooking and let it cool more quickly, put it in a salad bowl with a drizzle of oil to prevent it from sticking, mix it and put it in the fridge for about 20 minutes.

PASTA WITH BOTTARGA WITH FRESH TOMATO

Execution: easy

Time: 5 minutes + 10

Average cost

Ingredients for 4 people:

350 g of penne

60 g of bottarga

450 g of firm, ripe tomatoes

1 clove of garlic

3 sprigs of fresh basil

extra virgin olive oil to taste

chili pepper to taste salt to taste

Preparation

some penne with bottarga and fresh tomato,
How to blanch tomatoes in boiling water to
peel them easily Pour plenty of water into a
large pot, cover with the lid, heat it and, when
it boils, dip the tomatoes and blanch them for
1 minute. Then drain them (without throwing
away the hot water), pass them under running
tap water and remove the skin. Bring the
same water in which you blanched the
tomatoes back to the boil and, when it has
boiled again, add salt and add the pasta. In
the meantime, remove the peel from the garlic
clove, transfer it to a pan, add a drizzle of
extra virgin olive oil and a small piece of chilli
pepper without the seeds and fry briefly over
a low heat, stirring occasionally with a spoon
wooden.

Cut the tomatoes in half, remove the seeds, cut them into chunks and, as soon as the garlic begins to smell and take on a slightly golden colour, add them to the pan together with 1 tablespoon of basil leaves roughly chopped with your hands and cook for approximately 2 minutes. When the penne are cooked al dente, drain them, pour them into the pan, add the bottarga cut into thin flakes (or grated) and sauté everything, stirring delicately and adding a little cooking water if necessary. Remove the garlic clove, sprinkle with the remaining chopped basil off the heat, give it a final stir to mix the sauce well with the penne, plate it and, finally, immediately serve your delicious pasta with bottarga and fresh tomato.

LINGUINE WITH WALNUT PESTO, PINE NUTS AND MINT

Execution: very easy

Time: 5 minutes

+ 10 minutes of cooking

Cost: low

Ingredients for 4 people:

360 g of linguine

110 g of shelled walnuts

30 g of shelled and peeled pine nuts

80 g of grated parmesan

4 tablespoons of extra virgin olive oil

fresh mint to taste salt to taste

Preparation

Quick linguine with walnut pesto and mint pine nuts First, put a large pot with plenty of water on the heat. While the pasta cooking water heats up, prepare the walnut and pine nut pesto in this way: wash the mint leaves and dry them well (keeping some of them whole); place them in the blender glass together with the walnut kernels, pine nuts and any peeled and chopped garlic; operate the appliance; add the oil little by little and finally the grated parmesan and a pinch of salt. The sauce is ready: transfer it to a bowl and set it aside. When the water has reached the boil, add salt and add the pasta, adding a drizzle of oil to prevent it from sticking. Drain it just al dente, add the sauce and, if this is too thick for your tastes, dilute it in a little pasta cooking water.

CREAM OF PEAS AND SPRING ONIONS

Execution: easy

Time: 10 minutes

+ 12 minutes of cooking

Low price

Ingredients for 4 people:

4 cups fresh shelled peas

2 fresh spring onions

1 clove of garlic

1/2 cup fresh tarragon leaves

3 of EVO oil

1 1/2 liters of vegetable broth

toasted pistachios to taste

Salt and pepper to taste

Preparation

Spring onion bulbs and stems cut into rounds. Clean the spring onions, removing the roots at the base and the leaves but not the firm, greenish stems attached to the bulbs; wash them under running water to remove any residual soil, dry them and cut them first in half lengthwise and then into slices. Put the extra virgin olive oil in a large saucepan over a low heat and, as soon as it starts to foam, add the spring onions and the peeled garlic clove. Cover with the lid and cook for about ten minutes on a low heat, stirring often to prevent the vegetables from browning or, even worse, sticking to the bottom (if necessary, add a little boiling water). Once the spring onions have become soft, pour in 1 liter of boiling water

Pour in the broth, raise the heat and, when it comes to the boil again, add the shelled peas, season with the tarragon, lower the heat and continue cooking for 1012 minutes. When the peas have taken on a tender consistency, blend everything with the immersion blender until you obtain a smooth cream of the desired density. Season the pea and spring onion cream with salt and pepper, heat it briefly, keeping it on the heat for a few more minutes. If it is too liquid and needs to thicken, transfer it into individual bowls, decorate with toasted croutons or toasted pistachios and, finally, serve it on the table.

LIGHT SPINACH CREAM

Execution: easy

Time: 10 minutes

+15 minutes of cooking

Low price

Ingredients for 4 people:

1 kg of spinach;

1 clove of garlic

2 teaspoons of granulates

vegetable stock cube + 2 to prepare

any vegetable broth

4 tablespoons of cooking cream

extra virgin olive oil to taste

Salt and pepper to taste

Preparation

If you do not use already washed and trimmed spinach in a bag, clean it by eliminating the final part with the help of a sharp knife, wash it well with cold water to eliminate impurities and any soil remaining between the tufts, washing it several times if necessary . Once this is done, place them in a colander and let them drain. Remove the skin from the garlic clove, place it in a large saucepan, add a drizzle of EVO oil, and heat it over a low heat to prevent the garlic from browning and giving the dish a strong flavour. After 23 minutes, remove the garlic, add the spinach, the granular walnut and 2 glasses of boiling water, cover with the lid and cook for about fifteen minutes. Then turn off the heat, transfer the spinach with its cooking liquid into the blender glass and start blending it intermittently.

Then add 4 tablespoons of cream and continue
blending until you obtain a smooth soup of the
desired consistency, adding hot vegetable
broth if you want it more fluid, then season
with freshly ground pepper and taste to see if
the broth has made it savory enough or if you
have to salt it. Divide the spinach cream into
individual cups, drizzle each portion with a
drizzle of raw extra virgin olive oil and serve
this light but tasty first course hot.

THAI STYLE SHRIMP, MUSHROOM AND ASPARAGUS SOUP

Execution: easy

Time: 15 minutes

+ 15 minutes of cooking

Average cost

Ingredients for 4 people:

12 prawns, 12 asparagus

4 mushrooms

1 clove of garlic

1 untreated lemon

23 red chillies

the fresh, non-spicy kind

40 g of fresh ginger

1 teaspoon soy sauce

1 vegetable stock cube

Preparation

a little prawn, asparagus and mushroom soup according to the traditional Thai recipe. First you need to clean the prawns as follows: remove their carapace, keeping the tail attached; extract the black intestinal fillet from the dorsal part and eliminate it; rinse them under cold running water and then drain them. Remove the ginger peel, slice it and keep it aside. Clean the mushrooms, dry them with a soft cloth to remove dust and any other impurities present on their surface, cut them into thin slices, and sprinkle them with a small amount of filtered lemon juice. Place a saucepan with 1 liter of water on the heat and, when it comes to the boil, add the vegetable stock cube, a lemon zest, the peeled garlic and the ginger. When the stock cube has completely melted, pass the broth obtained through a sieve to filter it, leave in a few pieces of ginger and, if desired, the garlic, and transfer everything into a large pan. Bring back to the boil, and add the asparagus previously washed and cut into cubes, the mushrooms and peppers cut into strips. Wait a few minutes and then add the prawns and cook for about 5 minutes. Season the prawn, asparagus and mushroom soup with the soy sauce and the remaining lemon juice, season it, if you like, with a pinch of chilli powder as is often done in Thailand, and serve immediately.

ROASTED TOMATO CREAM

Execution: easy

Time: 10 minutes

+ 30 minutes of cooking

Low price

Ingredients for 4 people:

700 g of firm, ripe tomatoes

1 red chili pepper (optional)

1 onion, 1 clove of garlic

1 tablespoon balsamic vinegar

extra virgin olive oil to taste

oregano to taste

grated parmesan to taste

Salt and pepper to taste

Preparation

a little roasted tomato cream Wash the tomatoes, dry them and cut them into 2 or 4 pieces; peel the onion and cut it into wedges. Remove the stem from the pepper, cut it in half, remove the seeds and internal white ribs and cut it into not too thin layers. Arrange the vegetables on a baking tray without overlapping them, add the peeled garlic clove, season with EVO oil, salt and pepper, season with oregano, put in the oven and cook everything at 200° for about 30 minutes. Roasted tomatoes in the blender, Once the vegetables are roasted, transfer them to the blender glass, add the balsamic vinegar and blend them intermittently, adding a little boiling water at a time and in the quantity necessary to obtain the desired consistency, until obtaining a smooth cream. Divide the roasted tomato cream into individual bowls, add 1 tablespoon of yogurt to each if you serve it cold or 1 tablespoon of grated parmesan if you serve it hot or warm, season with a drizzle of oil, sprinkle with more if you like oregano and bring it to the table.

VEGETARIAN AND DIETARY

CORSE SOUP

Ingredients for 4 people:

2 stalks of celery

3 medium potatoes

1 onion

1 leek

120 grams of cabbage

2 cloves of garlic

1 vegetable stock cube

1 bunch of basil

4 slices of homemade bread

extra virgin olive oil to taste

Salt and pepper to taste

Preparation

quick vegetarian Corsican soup, peel the vegetables, remove: the skin and the ends of the carrots; celery filaments; the green part of the leek; the peel of potatoes, onion and garlic. Then wash them, drain them and cut them into small pieces, keeping aside 1 peeled and one whole clove of garlic. Coarsely cut the cabbage into small pieces or strips, rinse it under running water and drain it too. Heat 1 liter of water and dissolve the vegetable stock cube in it. Season all the vegetables with a drizzle of EVO oil in a high-sided saucepan for a few minutes, mixing them with a wooden spoon, then add the boiling broth and a pinch of salt.

Cook everything over medium heat (add more broth if necessary) and, in the meantime, toast the slices of bread, rub them with garlic and place one on the bottom of each bowl. Once the vegetables are cooked, taste and adjust salt and pepper to your taste. Pour the soup onto the bread into individual bowls, sprinkle with the washed, dried and roughly chopped basil leaves, add a drizzle of extra virgin olive oil and serve piping hot.

FRENCH ONION SOUP

Ingredients for 4 people:

4 large onions (1 kilo)

100 grams of gruyere

50 grams of butter

40 grams of white flour

1 liter of meat broth

1 bay leaf

1 glass of dry white wine

4 slices of homemade bread

Salt and pepper to taste

Preparation

of white onion soup au gratin according to the French recipe. Prepare the meat broth at home or, if you want to use less time, do it with the stock cube as follows: put a saucepan with 1 liter of water on the heat; add the diced meat as soon as it starts to boil; lower the heat and continue to cook until the concentrate cube has completely dissolved. Onions should be cut into thin slices to make soup. Clean the onions, wash them, dry them, cut them into thin slices, place them in a saucepan, and cook them in the butter over a low heat for about fifteen minutes, stirring often with a wooden spoon and wetting them with half the white wine. How to brown the onions for the soup When the onions have "sweated" and become transparent and slightly blonde without having taken on a dark color anywhere, sprinkle them with the sifted flour, mix delicately for a few minutes to incorporate it well and mix with the remaining wine.

of broth and simmer for about 3040 minutes over low heat, adding the remaining broth little by little to ensure that it does not thicken too much, before salting and peppering the onion cream obtained. In the meantime, heat the oven to 200°, cut the homemade bread into 4 slices, place them in the oven, and toast them, being careful not to burn them; Pass the Gruyere cheese on the side with the larger holes and keep it aside. Cut each slice of bread into 2 parts and arrange 1 on the bottom of 4 small individual baking dishes, pour over 2 ladles of white onion soup and sprinkle with the grated Gruyere cheese. Make an equal layer with the remaining slice, more broth and more cheese, and season with freshly ground pepper before transferring the dishes into the hot oven and gratinating at 200° for a few minutes until the cheese has completely melted and took on a golden color. Serve the steaming soupe à l'oignon on the table.

SPAGHETTI WITH RANCETTO

Execution: easy

Time: 10 minutes

+ 20 minutes of cooking

Low price

Ingredients for 4 people:

400 g of spaghetti

1 200 g slice of bacon

40 g of grated pecorino

1 white onion

600 g of peeled tomatoes

1 sprig of marjoram

extra virgin olive oil to taste

black pepper to taste salt to taste

Preparation

First, cut the bacon into equal pieces and clean the onion, wash it, dry it and chop it finely. Pour 1 drizzle of extra virgin olive oil into a pan, add the pieces of bacon and brown them over low heat for 5 minutes, stirring occasionally with a wooden spoon. In the meantime, put a pan with plenty of water on the heat to cook the pasta. When the bacon cubes are golden on the surface, remove them from the pan and season the chopped onion with the fat released by them over a medium heat. As soon as the onion is golden, add the chopped tomatoes, put the lid on and continue cooking for about ten minutes before removing the pan from the heat and adding the chopped marjoram, salt, and freshly ground pepper. The water in the pan will start to boil, add salt, add the pasta and boil until it is al dente. Then drain it, pour it into the pan containing the sauce, add the bacon, and mix everything well, adding a little cooking water if necessary. Then turn off the heat, sprinkle generously with the grated pecorino, mix again, divide the spaghetti with the rancetto into individual plates, drizzle each with a drizzle of raw oil and serve piping hot.

CUCUMBER SPAGHETTI WITH TOMATOES, BASIL AND OLIVES

Difficulty: easy 35 minutes

ingredients

For 4 people

1.5 kg of cucumbers

400 g of cherry tomatoes

60 g of pitted black olives

1 tablespoon chopped chives

10 Basil leaves

1 piece of fresh chilli

2 tablespoons extra virgin olive oil

2 tablespoons of apple cider vinegar

Salt, pepper, oregano

Preparation

Peel the cucumbers, or leave the peel if it is not particularly thick, then cut them into spaghetti with the appropriate tool. In the absence of the latter, use a potato peeler to first divide them into many thin ribbons and then into tagliatelle (in this case discard the most watery part with the seeds). Season the cucumbers with vinegar and a pinch of salt, mix them well and leave them to marinate in the refrigerator for at least 20 minutes. Cut the cherry tomatoes into small pieces, then chop the basil and chilli pepper with a knife, adjusting the quantity according to personal taste. Season the tomatoes with chopped basil and chilli pepper, chives and chopped olives, salt, pepper and oregano. Drain the cucumber spaghetti (or tagliatelle) and squeeze them gently. In a salad bowl,

TAGLIATELLE IN CREAM BROCCOLETTI AND WALNUTS WITH POCHÈ EGGS

Difficulty: easy

Time 5 minutes +15 minutes

ingredients

For 4 people

300 g of dry egg pasta

4 eggs

300 g of broccoli

12 walnut kernels

3 tablespoons grated parmesan

Half lemons

extra virgin olive oil

Salt and pepper

Preparation

Dip the florets in a large pan of boiling salted water. Then boil them for about 8 minutes or until soft. Drain them with a slotted spoon, keeping the water aside, and let them cool. Keep a few florets aside for decoration and blend the rest with the juice and zest of half a lemon, 23 tablespoons of oil, salt, pepper, walnuts and parmesan. Gradually pour in enough water until you obtain the consistency of a creamy pesto. Pour the tagliatelle into the boiling water with the florets. At the same time, prepare the poached eggs, one at a time. Break the first one into a small bowl and pour it into a pan of lightly salted boiling water after creating a small vortex in the centre. Cook until the egg white has set around the yolk

(about 2 minutes) which will remain soft.
Drain it gently with a slotted spoon onto a
plate. Proceed with the remaining eggs. In a
bowl, dissolve the cream with a little pasta
cooking water. Then drain the tagliatelle,
stirring vigorously to season them evenly.
Distribute the pasta onto plates and decorate
with the florets kept aside. Place an egg in the
center, picking it up delicately with a spoon,
then season it with a pinch of salt and pepper.
Complete with a drizzle of oil, a sprinkling of
parmesan and serve.

BUCKWHEAT WITH VEGETABLES AND CHESTNUTS WITH CREAM OF RED CABBAGE

Difficulty: easy 30 minutes

ingredients

For 4 people

200 g of buckwheat grains

500 g red cabbage

400 g of broccoli

300 g Pumpkin pulp

12 Chestnuts, 8 Walnuts

2 peppers, 2 bay leaves

1 teaspoon of rosemary

1 chili pepper, salt

extra virgin olive oil

Preparation

Cut the chestnuts and boil them in plenty of water with the bay leaf for 20/25 minutes. Then peel them and cut them into pieces. Gently toast the buckwheat for 23 minutes in a heavy-bottomed saucepan, then pour in half a liter of hot water and bring to the boil. Add salt and partially cover the pan with a lid, then cook for 15 minutes over low heat. Remove from the heat and leave to rest for 5/10 minutes. Fry the peppers in 4 tablespoons of very hot oil for 5/10 seconds maximum, until they are crispy but be careful not to burn them. Drain them from the oil and, once cold, divide them into small pieces. Cut the pumpkin into cubes, and season it with the rosemary, 2 tablespoons of pepper oil and a little salt.

Spread it on a baking tray lined with baking paper and bake at 180°C for 15 minutes. Divide the broccoli into florets and steam them for about 10 minutes. Coarsely chop the cabbage and season it with the remaining oil from the peppers, a pinch of salt and the chilli pepper. Cook it in a saucepan for 15‑20 minutes, pouring in a little water. Blend until you obtain a cream. Mix the buckwheat with the chestnuts, broccoli, pumpkin, peppers and chopped walnuts, arrange it in the shape of a donut on the plates and place the cream in the centre.

MALTAGLIATI WITH LEEKS AND OF MUSHROOMS AND HAZELNUTS SAUCE

Difficulty: easy

Time 60 minutes +35 minutes

ingredients

For 4 people

400 g re-milled durum wheat semolina

400 g of leeks, 300 g of mixed mushrooms

40 g Hazelnuts, 1 clove Garlic

1 handful of parsley

1 dried chilli, 25 g butter

40 g grated parmesan

extra virgin olive oil

Salt, pepper, paprika

Preparation

Peel the leeks, set aside 2 cm of the whitest part and slice the rest into thin slices. Heat 2 tablespoons of oil in a pan, add the leeks and simmer over medium heat for 10 minutes. Then blend them with 150 ml of water until you obtain a smooth cream. Mix half a teaspoon of salt with the semolina and arrange it in a mound on a pastry board. Pour the blended leeks into the center and knead vigorously until you obtain a compact and elastic dough, adding more water or semolina if necessary. Form a ball, cover it and let it rest for about an hour. Prepare the dressing. Finely chop the garlic and leek kept aside, then brown them gently in a pan with 2 tablespoons of oil and the whole chilli pepper.

At this point add the coarsely chopped hazelnuts and the chopped parsley. Cook for a couple of minutes, then remove the chilli. Add the cleaned and diced mushrooms. Sauté them over high heat for 45 minutes, then blend them with the Marsala. Continue for 15 minutes, adding salt and pepper towards the end. Roll out the dough, on a surface dusted with more semolina, into sheets of about 2 mm thick. With the serrated wheel, cut out lozenges a couple of fingers wide, placing them gradually in a cardboard tray or in a cloth lightly dusted with semolina. Boil the maltagliati for 2 minutes in plenty of salted water, stirring often to prevent them from sticking together. Drain them and let them flavor for a couple of minutes in the pan with the mushrooms, adding the cold butter from the fridge and the parmesan to mix everything together.

**PISTACHIO GNOCCHI
IN PUMPKIN SAUCE**

Time 10 minutes

Difficulty: Medium

ingredients

For 6 people

1.3 kg White pulp potatoes

300 g type 00 soft wheat flour

Nutmeg

Salt, oil

250 g of pumpkin

150 g of pistachios

80 g of scamorza

1 leek, 1 tablespoon of parsley

0.5 cloves of garlic

Preparation

Proceed as for traditional gnocchi and prepare the dough. Once ready, combine the blended pistachios and the finely chopped parsley with the garlic. Peel and finely slice the leek, brown it for 10 minutes together with 4 tablespoons of oil, add the diced pumpkin, salt, cover and continue cooking for 1520 minutes over medium-low heat. Blend it, diluting it with a few tablespoons of hot water until you obtain a fairly fluid sauce. Boil the gnocchi, drain them, place them on plates and cover them with the sauce and the coarsely grated scamorza.

CHESTNUT TAGLIOLINI WITH LEEKS IN RED WINE AND ALMONDS

Difficulty: Easy

30 minutes + 25 minutes

ingredients

For 4 people

200 g of flour

50 g of chestnut flour

2 eggs, 4 leeks

60 g Almonds

1 teaspoon chopped parsley

1 sprig of Rosemary

400ml Red wine

Extra virgin olive oil, pepper, salt

Preparation

Mix the white flour with the chestnut flour, then arrange them in a well and knead them for a long time together with a pinch of salt, ground pepper, the eggs and the water needed to obtain a smooth dough. Cover it and let it rest for an hour. Finely chop the rosemary needles together with a third of the almonds and mix them immediately with 45 tablespoons of oil. Slice the leeks as thinly as possible, then season them with a pinch of salt and the rosemary oil and brown them in a pan with the lid on for 15 minutes over medium-low heat. After this time, pour in the wine, raise the heat and let it reduce to a third of the initial dose.

Toast the remaining almonds over low heat in a saucepan for 5 minutes, stirring often. Let them cool and chop them. Roll out the dough to a height of about 4 mm and cut out the tagliolini. Boil them for 23 minutes in plenty of salted water, drain them while they are not too dry and transfer them to the pan with the leeks, sautéing them for a few seconds over a high heat. Finally add the parsley and almonds, mix and serve.

EGG TAGLIOLINI WITH LENTIL RAGU AND PORCINI MUSHROOMS

Difficulty: Easy

Time 10 minutes + 20 minutes

ingredients

For 4 people

250 g dried lentils, cooked

220 g fresh pasta cutters

200 g Tomatoes, pureed

2 porcini mushrooms

20 g Dried porcini mushrooms

4 teaspoons of grated parmesan

1 stick of celery

1 carrot, 0.5 onion

1 sprig of Rosemary

Extra virgin olive oil

Salt and pepper

Preparation

Soak the dried mushrooms in 130 ml of hot water for about ten minutes. Cut the carrot, celery and onion into small cubes and brown them in a pan with 2 tablespoons of oil together with the rosemary. At this point add the well-squeezed soaked mushrooms, filter the soaking water and use about half of it to blend the vegetables. Clean the fresh porcini mushrooms, slice them and add them to the pan with the vegetables; leave to flavor for 5 minutes and then blend with the rest

the water from soaking the dried mushrooms.
Add the lentils and after a while the tomato
puree. Add salt and pepper and continue on a
high heat for 15 minutes, stirring occasionally.
Boil the tagliolini in plenty of lightly salted
water for about 4 minutes. Drain them
(reserve a little water in case you need it to
make everything softer), then season them
with the lentil sauce and a drizzle of oil.
Distribute them on plates and complete them
with parmesan.

BREAD PIZZAS WITH LEEKS, BRIE AND HAZELNUTS

Difficulty: easy

Time 20 minutes +30 minutes

ingredients

For 6 people

350 g stale bread

3 leeks

200 g of brie

50 g of toasted hazelnuts

6 sprigs of thyme

extra virgin olive oil

Salt and pepper

Preparation

Tear the bread into a bowl with your hands or a knife, depending on its hardness. Separately, emulsify 200 ml of water with 50 ml of oil, then add them little by little to the bowl, kneading and crumbling the bread. Once all the emulsion has been incorporated, work for a few more seconds, always breaking the bread into pieces, until the mixture has taken the shape of a coarse dough. Let it rest for 10 minutes. Cut the leeks into slices about one centimeter thick and simmer them over medium-low heat in a pan with 23 tablespoons of oil for 10 minutes. Halfway through cooking, add a little salt, pepper and the leaves of 3 sprigs of thyme. Remove from the heat and blend half the leeks, keeping the rest aside.

Brush a 24x28 cm pan with one or two tablespoons of oil and distribute the mixture inside, compacting it very well with your hands, without leaving spaces. Add the leek cream, spreading it on the edges too, then arrange the remaining leeks, and a little bits of brie (cutting the rest into slices for decoration), and complete with a drizzle of oil. Bake the pizza at 180°C for about 15 minutes. After this time, add the chopped hazelnuts and the leaves of the remaining thyme sprigs. Then move the pan to the lowest part of the oven, in direct contact: this way it will become crispier. Remove it after about 5 minutes, garnish it with the slices of brie and serve hot.

SAFFRON TAGLIOLINI IN FRESH LEEK AND PORCINI CREAM

Difficulty: medium

Time 45 minutes + 30 minutes

ingredients

For 4 people

200 g of 0 flour

100 g of durum wheat semolina

3 eggs, 400 g of porcini mushrooms

120 g of white pulp potatoes

2 leeks, 1 clove of garlic

1 sprig of Rosemary

1 sachet of saffron, 100 ml of milk, salt

extra virgin olive oil

Preparation

Mix the flour with the semolina and a pinch of salt, then form the classic fountain on the pastry board. Pour the eggs already beaten with the saffron into the center and gradually add the necessary water to obtain a soft dough to cover and leave to rest for 30 minutes. Chop the garlic together with the rosemary needles. Then clean the porcini mushrooms and slice them finely. In a pan, brown the chopped garlic briefly with 23 tablespoons of oil and add the mushrooms, salt them, then cover them with the lid and cook them for 10 minutes over medium heat. After this time, drain the mushrooms from the pan, strengthen the bottom with a drizzle of oil and brown the thinly sliced leeks over medium-low heat for about ten minutes.

Peel and dice the potatoes, then boil them in salted water for 5 minutes, drain them with a slotted spoon (reserve their water) directly into the fried leeks together with a third of the sautéed mushrooms. Continue for another 5 minutes and blend everything with the necessary milk to obtain a creamy sauce. Finally check the salt. Roll out the dough to a thickness of 34 mm and then cut out the tagliolini. Boil them in boiling potato water and drain them not too dry in a bowl, seasoning them immediately with a drizzle of oil. Distribute the pasta on the plates, place the sauce in the center and place the remaining sautéed mushrooms on top, possibly decorating with saffron pistils.

PINK RICOTTA AND BEETROOT GNOCCHI WITH SAGE

Difficulty: Easy

Time 25 minutes + 10 minutes

For 4 people

ingredients

125 g white flour

80 g breadcrumbs

2 eggs, 350 g of ricotta

2 tablespoons grated parmesan

60 g Red beets, cooked

20 Sage leaf

1 tablespoon poppy seeds

Extra virgin olive oil

Salt and pepper

Preparation

Beat the eggs with a little salt and pepper, the breadcrumbs and the blended and creamed beetroot; add the ricotta and, after kneading it, add the flour and parmesan until a soft, dry dough forms (if it is still too soft, add more flour). Take one dough at a time with floured hands and cut it into small round dumplings to place on a floured tray. Toast the poppy seeds in a pan for 23 minutes, set them aside and in the same pan heat 45 tablespoons of oil over a low heat for 23 minutes with the sage leaves. Boil the gnocchi in plenty of salted water for about 5 minutes, drain them with a slotted spoon. directly into the pan with the oil and let them flavor briefly, completing with the poppy seeds.

BARLEY AND BORLOTTI BEAN SALAD IN YOGURT SAUCE

Difficulty: easy

Time 20 minutes + 30 minutes

Ingredients for 4 people

250 g of pearl barley

200 g of cooked borlotti beans

150 g of cherry tomatoes, 10 cashews

4 walnuts, 20 g of pine nuts

1 bunch of parsley

Salt, For the sauce

125 g low-fat yogurt

10 stems of chives

extra virgin olive oil

sweet paprika, salt

Preparation

Rinse the barley well under running water, then cook it in plenty of lightly salted water for about 30 minutes. Once ready, drain it and spread it on a tray to cool. Cut the cherry tomatoes into 4 wedges; then toast the pine nuts in a fat-free pan for 34 minutes over a low heat. Finally, coarsely chop the walnuts and cashews. It's time to prepare the sauce by blending the yogurt with the chopped chives, 2 tablespoons of oil, a sprinkling of paprika and salt. Now compose the dish by combining the barley, beans, chopped cashews and walnuts, pine nuts, cherry tomatoes and coarsely chopped parsley, including the stems, in a bowl. All you have to do is mix the sauce and the salad is ready to be enjoyed.

BUTTERFLIES WITH THY ME SCENTED PEPPERS

Difficulty: Easy

Time 20 minutes +30 minutes

ingredients

For 4 people

320 g of farfalle pasta

2 peppers, red

200 grams of courgettes

200 g of ricotta

100ml Milk

4 spring onions

1 bunch of thyme

Oil, pepper, salt

Preparation

Peel the spring onions, keeping most of the green leaves and slice them finely. Remove the stem and seeds from the peppers and cut them into cubes. Cut the courgettes into slightly larger cubes. Fry the spring onions in 34 tablespoons of oil for 10 minutes in a large pan over medium-low heat. Add the peppers and courgettes, add salt, cover, lower the heat and continue cooking for another 15 minutes. In the meantime, peel the thyme and put it in a blender together with the ricotta, milk, ground pepper and a little salt. Blend everything until you obtain a fragrant and homogeneous sauce. Add the sauce to the vegetables, cook for another minute and add salt if necessary. Boil the farfalle al dente, drain them while not too dry, add them to the pan with the vegetables and serve immediately.

SPAGHETTI WITH GREEN BEANS, BASIL AND CHILI PEPPER

Difficulty: easy

Time 10 minutes 15 minutes

ingredients

For 4 people

Spaghetti 320 g

500 g of green beans

1 bunch Basil

1 lemon, salt, 1 clove of garlic

extra virgin olive oil

Dried chili flakes

Preparation

Finely chop the garlic and brown it over a very low heat in a large pan (where you want it).

then sauté the pasta) with 45 tablespoons of oil and a pinch of chilli pepper. Remove the pan from the heat and keep it aside. Bring a pan of lightly salted water to the boil and add the pasta and green beans, already peeled and cut into 2 parts. Cook for about 2 minutes less than the time indicated on the spaghetti package. Put the pan with the garlic back on the heat and pour in a ladle of the pasta water. Drain the spaghetti with the green beans (reserving a full glass of the cooking water) and transfer them to the pan. Then cook them, adding a little of their water, when the previous one has been absorbed, in order to bind the pasta to the sauce. Also add the coarsely chopped basil and a splash of lemon juice. Complete the spaghetti, away from the heat, with a generous grate of lemon zest, a drizzle of oil,

**SMALL WARM TIMBALES
WITH AUBERGINES
AND OLIVES**

Difficulty: Easy

Time 60 minutes 40 minutes

ingredients

For 4 people

250 g Pasta Ditalini rigati

500 g cherry tomatoes

3 aubergines

100 g Olives, 40 g Pecorino

2 tablespoons pine nuts

1 shallot, 1 chilli pepper

Basil, Oil, Salt

Chilli powder

Preparation

Cut the aubergines into half-centimeter thick slices lengthwise, and cook them for 67 minutes on a grill or in a greased pan, turning them only once. Finely chop the shallot and gently brown it in 4 tablespoons of oil. Add the chili pepper, sliced tomatoes, salt, put the lid on and cook for about a quarter of an hour. Finally remove the pepper. Pass the sauce obtained through a sieve, pour it back into the pan and cook for 5 minutes so that it thickens. Add the chopped basil, most of the pitted and chopped olives (keep a dozen aside), and the pine nuts previously toasted in a saucepan.

Finally check the salt. Boil the pasta in plenty of salted water, drain it al dente and stop cooking with a little cold water, season it with the sauce and crumbled pecorino cheese. Cover 4 small bowls with a diameter of 10 cm with cling film and lightly grease them; cover them with the aubergine slices, fill them with the pasta and close them with the remaining aubergine slices. Seal each with cling film and leave to rest for 20/30 minutes.

SPELLED PENNETTE WITH PARMESAN AND RATATUJA

Difficulty: Easy

Time 25 minutes + 30 minutes

ingredients

For 4 people

300 g spelled penne

2 potatoes, 2 carrots

4 courgettes, 1 spring onion

1 clove of garlic, 4 copper tomatoes

1 handful of basil, 1 tablespoon of parsley

4 tablespoons of extra virgin olive oil

1 pinch of chilli powder

40 g parmesan, salt

Preparation

After washing and cleaning them, cut the carrots, potatoes and courgettes into cubes of the same size. Keep them separate. Heat two tablespoons of oil in a non-stick pan and brown the peeled and chopped garlic and spring onion. Add the chopped parsley, carrots and potatoes, cover and cook for about 78 minutes over low heat, then add the courgettes and continue cooking for another 1215 minutes. Add salt according to your taste. Blanch the tomatoes in a little boiling water. Peel them, let them cool, and cut them into cubes of the same size as you cut the other vegetables.

Add them to the rest of the vegetables just before turning off, season with salt, and add the basil chopped with your hands. Cook the pasta, drain it al dente, and pour it into the pan together with the vegetables, to which you will also add a couple of spoons of its cooking water. Complete with a drizzle of extra virgin olive oil and brown over high heat in a large non-stick pan for 2 minutes. Serve hot, sprinkled with flakes of medium-aged parmesan and a sprinkling of chilli pepper, adjusting according to your tastes.

SPAGHETTI WITH DOUBLE TOMATO WITH BASIL

Difficulty: easy

Time 25 minutes

ingredients

For 4 people

280 g Spaghetti

350 grams of tomatoes

15 cherry tomatoes

4 tablespoons of breadcrumbs

2 tablespoons grated parmesan

1 teaspoon Capers

1 clove Garlic

10 parsley leaves

Basil salt

extra virgin olive oil

Preparation

Prepare a filling by finely chopping half a clove of garlic, the capers, the parsley and 2 basil leaves, mix in the breadcrumbs, parmesan and lightly salt. Cut the cherry tomatoes in half, remove the seeds and place them in a baking dish with the cut side facing up. Fill them with the filling, drizzle them with a drizzle of oil and bake at 180°C for 1015 minutes or until they are golden brown. Heat 2 tablespoons of oil in a large pan, and add the remaining half clove of garlic, the cherry tomatoes ox heart cut into cubes, lightly salt and sauté over high heat for 2 minutes.

Wash off the heat and mix in 3 chopped basil leaves. Let its flavor. Boil the spaghetti al dente, drain them and pour them into the pan with the chopped tomatoes removed from the garlic, sauté them for one to two minutes, allowing them to flavor well, then distribute them on the plates. Complete the dish with gratin cherry tomatoes, a few chopped basil leaves and possibly more parmesan to taste. Spaghetti seasoned in this way is excellent served both hot and warm.

POTATO GNOCCHI WITH PEAS AND BASIL VEGETABLES

Difficulty: easy

Time 10 minutes + 25 minutes

ingredients

For 4 people

800 g Potato gnocchi

300 g of fresh shelled peas

3 courgettes, 2 spring onions

30 g of unpeeled almonds

1 clove Garlic

1 bunch of basil, 1 lemon

extra virgin olive oil

Dried chili pepper, salt and pepper

Preparation

Thinly slice the spring onions, including some of the green part. Finely chop the garlic. Put them both to stew in a pan with 2 tablespoons of oil over very low heat, without letting them brown; if necessary, add a little water. Once wilted, mix the peas with the herbs and cook for 12 minutes, adding a little water from time to time if necessary. Peel the courgettes, divide them in half lengthwise and slice them quite finely. Then add them to the peas and continue cooking for another 5 minutes. Finally, season with salt and pepper and add the finely chopped basil leaves. Get out of the fire.

Toast the almonds in a pan over low heat. Once cooled, chop them as finely as possible. Cut many thin strips from the lemon zest. Dip the gnocchi in lightly salted boiling water and drain them with a slotted spoon (save the cooking water) when they come to the surface, transferring them to the pan with the peas. Sauté the gnocchi over high heat with the sauce for about a minute, pouring a ladle of their water until a creamy and enveloping sauce is formed. Arrange the gnocchi on plates and complete them with lemon zest, a pinch of chilli pepper and a sprinkling of chopped almonds.

ASPARAGUS LASAGNA

Difficulty: medium

Time 60 minutes + 45 minutes

ingredients

For 6 people

For pasta

300 g of 0 flour

8 asparagus

3 eggs, salt

For the stuffing

1 kg of asparagus,

150 g parmesan

2 shallots, 40 g of pine nuts,

Salt and pepper

Preparation

Mix the flour with the eggs and a pinch of salt until you obtain a very smooth and compact but still soft dough. Cover it with a cloth and let it rest for at least 30 minutes. Clean the asparagus for the pasta and slice them thinly lengthwise with a potato peeler. Roll out the slices and cover them to prevent them from curling. Remove the hardest parts of the asparagus for the filling and cut them into slices. Brown the chopped shallot with 2 tablespoons of oil for 5 minutes, then add the asparagus and toast them briefly. Salt and pepper and then add the pine nuts and half a glass of water. Cover with a lid and cook for about 10 minutes. Finally, blend a third of the vegetables to obtain a cream.

Roll out the dough finely with the appropriate tool and cut it into rectangles of approximately 14x10 cm. Place 3 slices of asparagus in the center of 2 overlapping rectangles of puff pastry and pass them through the machine to seal them very well. Repeat the operation for all sheets. Spread a drizzle of asparagus cream on the bottom of a 25 x 32 cm pan, then arrange a layer of puff pastry, a little cream and a little steamed asparagus, then sprinkle with grated parmesan. Repeat the operation and finish with the stewed asparagus and plenty of parmesan. Bake the lasagna at 180°C for about 25 minutes.

MEDITERRANEAN OVEN STUFFED ARTICHOKES

Difficulty: easy

Time 15 minutes + 25 minutes

ingredients

For 4 people

4 artichokes

2 slices of bread

2 tablespoons grated parmesan

1 lemon

1 clove Garlic

10 sprigs of parsley

1 tablespoon Capers

half a glass dry white wine

extra virgin olive oil

Coarse salt, fine salt, pepper

Preparation

Bring the water to the boil in a saucepan with the white wine and a pinch of coarse salt. Clean the artichokes, remove the toughest leaves and the stem, then cut them at the base so that they remain vertical. Clean the base of the artichokes and the tender part of the stems with a small knife, then rub them with the lemon cut in half. Then cut 2 pieces of zest from the lemon which you will need for the filling. Spread the artichokes in the center with your hands and with a small spatula remove the beard, keeping them whole. Rinse them and immerse them in boiling water together with the peeled stems.

Boil them for 12 minutes, then drain them and let them cool in cold water to stop the cooking. Chop the bread into small pieces in the mixer until it is reduced to rather small crumbs. Place the bread in a bowl and then combine the parsley leaves, garlic, previously desalted capers and 2 pieces of lemon zest in the mixer. Chop until you obtain a fine mixture and then mix it with the bread, then add the parmesan, 2 tablespoons of oil, salt and pepper. Mix with a fork, fluffing the bread to obtain coarse crumbs. Stuff the artichokes with the aromatic mixture, place them together with the stems in a pan lightly greased with oil, and place them in the oven at 200°C in ventilated mode for 1012 minutes or until the bread is golden on the surface. Let them cool before serving.

GREEN LINGUINE WITH SPINACH AND GOAT'S RICOTTA

Difficulty: easy

Time 10 minutes + 15 minutes

ingredients

For 4 people

320 g wholemeal linguine

100 g Spinach

200 g goat's ricotta

50 g parmesan

extra virgin olive oil

Salt and pepper optional

Preparation

Dip the linguine in a pan of boiling salted water, mix and place the spinach on the surface, which will simply have to dry for 2 minutes. Take them out with a slotted spoon, or with kitchen tongs, and put them directly into the blender. Blend the spinach with the ricotta, 23 tablespoons of oil, a sprinkling of salt and, if necessary, pepper. Drain the linguine al dente in a bowl, keeping aside a ladle of their water. Season them immediately with the green cream, adding a little cooking water if necessary, then stir in half the grated parmesan. Divide the pasta between plates, sprinkle with the remaining cheese and serve immediately.

**TURNIP SPATZLE
WITH PINE NUTS**

Difficulty: easy

Time 15 minutes + 15 minutes

ingredients

For 4 people

Spatzle 320 g

400 g turnip greens

50 g pine nuts

50 g wholemeal breadcrumbs

2 cloves of garlic

Extra virgin olive oil

Chilli powder

salt

Preparation

Peel and briefly blanch the turnip greens, drain them well, squeeze them and cut them with a pair of kitchen scissors. In a pan, gently toast the pine nuts and then add 23 tablespoons of oil, the turnip greens, the garlic cloves with their peel, a sprinkling of chilli pepper, and brown everything, leaving it to infuse. Finally remove the garlic. Boil the spätzle and drain them into the pan with the vegetables, mixing carefully. On the plates, if you want, complete with a sprinkling of breadcrumbs previously toasted in a pan and made crunchy.

**WHITE ARTICHOKES
AND WALNUT LASAGNA**

Difficulty: Easy

Time 20 minutes + 50 minutes

ingredients

For 4 people

250g Pasta for fresh egg lasagne

15 Artichokes

150 g of walnuts, 100 g of flour

100 g of butter, 1 l of milk

Extra virgin olive oil

pepper, salt, nutmeg

Preparation

Clean the artichokes, then divide each one into 8 segments which you will blanch in plenty of salted water for 78 minutes. Drain the

artichoke segments and season them in a pan with 23 tablespoons of oil, salt and pepper. Heat the butter in a pan, and gradually add the flour, stirring constantly until a biscuit aroma is released; at this point pour in all the cold milk and work vigorously with a whisk. Cook the béchamel until you obtain the desired consistency, seasoning it with salt, pepper and nutmeg. Chop the walnuts quickly in the blender, obtaining a rather coarse grain (it must not be greasy). Arrange the lasagna in a rectangular baking dish, alternating layers of pasta and bechamel sauce sprinkled with walnuts and artichokes. Finish with the béchamel sauce and decorate the surface with some chopped walnuts and a few artichoke segments. All you have to do is bake at 165°C for 40 minutes.

WHOLE BAVETTE WITH ARTICHOKES IN CURRY ONION SAUCE

Difficulty: Easy

Time 20 minutes + 40 minutes

Ingredients for 4 people

320 g wholemeal bavette,

200 g of ricotta

6 Artichokes, 3 Onions

1 tablespoon curry

0.5 lemon, 100 ml of milk

Vegetable broth

Extra virgin olive oil

Parsley, pink pepper, salt

Preparation

Cut the onions into thin wedges, season them with 23 tablespoons of oil, a pinch of salt and the curry, then brown them in a pan. Cover with a lid and continue over low heat for 1520 minutes, wetting the onions with broth or water only if necessary. Carefully clean the artichokes, and slice them finely by immersing them in water acidulated with lemon juice. Remove the onions from the pan, heat one or two tablespoons of oil and add the well-drained artichokes; salt them, then cover them with the lid and cook them for about ten minutes. Blend the onions with the ricotta and the necessary milk to obtain a rather fluid sauce. Finally check the salt and add more curry according to personal taste. Boil the bavette al dente, drain them not too dry directly into the artichoke pan and add the curry sauce. On the plates, sprinkle the pasta with chopped parsley and a few pink peppercorns.

PIZZOCCHERI WITH TOPINAMBUR AND CHICORY

Difficulty: easy

Time 20 minutes +15 minutes

ingredients

For 4 people

250 g of pizzoccheri

400 g of Jerusalem artichokes

400 g red chicory

100 g of fresh goat's cheese

4 sprigs of thyme

2 tablespoons extra virgin olive oil

Salt and pepper

Preparation

Peel and slice the radicchio rather thinly. Fry it in a pan with oil and thyme for about 5 minutes. Finally sprinkle it with salt and pepper. Peel the Jerusalem artichokes and cut them into cubes. Then boil them together with the pizzoccheri in plenty of boiling salted water. Bring to the boil and drain everything directly into the pan with the radicchio, keeping aside a glass of the pasta water. Mix the various ingredients well over a high heat, adding, if necessary, a little of the pizzoccheri cooking water. Remove the thyme sprigs and add the goat cheese, letting it melt. Remove from the heat and complete with freshly ground pepper on the plates.

TORTIGLIIONE CARBONARA

Difficulty: easy

Time 20 minutes + 25 minutes

ingredients

For 4 people

360 g Tortiglioni

800 g of mushrooms

2 eggs, 2 yolks

80 g parmesan

5 peeled cooked chestnuts

1 clove Garlic

8 sprigs of thyme

extra virgin olive oil

Salt and pepper

Preparation

Clean the mushrooms and divide them into 24 parts depending on their size (so as to obtain more or less equal pieces) and place them in a large pan without seasoning them. Sprinkle them with a pinch of salt and pepper and add the lightly crushed garlic. Cover with the lid and cook them over medium heat until they begin to release the vegetable water. Uncover the pan and let the bottom dry almost completely. At this point add 2 tablespoons of oil and sauté the mushrooms for 56 minutes, until they are golden but still slightly al dente. Check the salt and remove from the heat. In the meantime, bring a pan of lightly salted water to the boil and add the tortiglioni. While the pasta is cooking, combine all the eggs in a large bowl and grate them parmesan, plenty of freshly ground pepper, a pinch of salt and the leaves of the thyme sprigs. Mix carefully until you obtain a smooth cream. Then dilute it slightly by pouring very little pasta cooking water. Add the tortiglioni to the eggs, drain them with a slotted spoon (keep the water in the pan) and mix vigorously. Add the mushrooms, without the garlic, and mix well. If you notice that there is some liquid egg left on the bottom, place the bowl with the pasta in a bain-marie in the now turned off pasta water and stir until the sauce has thickened slightly. However, if it seems a little dry, soften it with a little cooking water. Divide the tortiglioni among the plates, distribute the sliced chestnuts on top and a final sprinkling of parmesan and pepper.

CREAMY ORECCHIETTE WITH PORCINI MUSHROOMS AND PARSLEY

Difficulty: easy

Time 10 minutes + 20 minutes

ingredients

For 4 people

400 g fresh Orecchiette

400 g of porcini mushrooms

120 gr Mascarpone

40 g parmesan

2 cloves Garlic

1 bunch of parsley

extra virgin olive oil

Salt and pepper

Preparation

Clean the porcini mushrooms and cut them into not too small segments, dividing only the smaller mushrooms in half. In a large non-stick pan, brown the sliced or chopped garlic together with 34 tablespoons of oil. Then add the mushrooms and brown them for about ten minutes. Just before removing from the heat, add salt and pepper and sprinkle with half the chopped parsley. Boil the orecchiette in abundant salted water and drain them al dente, keeping aside a ladle of their water. Place them in the pan with the mushrooms over a very low heat and stir in the mascarpone and the cooking water needed for a creamy result. Serve the pasta immediately, sprinkling it onto the plates with the grated parmesan, the rest of the parsley and, if desired, a sprinkling of pepper.

ROMAN-STYLE GNOCCHI WHITE WITH POLENTA WITH WALNUTS AND SAGE

Difficulty: medium

Time 10 minutes + 60 minutes

ingredients

For 4 people

250 g of white corn flour

100 g parmesan

100 g Pecorino

30 g of butter

3 tablespoons of walnut kernels

12 sage leaves

extra virgin olive oil

Coarse salt, pepper

Preparation

Bring one liter and 750 ml of water to the boil with a teaspoon of coarse salt. Mix the corn flour, bring to the boil, then reduce the heat to low and continue, stirring constantly, for about 50 minutes. At the end of cooking, mix together a sprinkling of pepper, the butter, the grated Parmesan and the pecorino, keeping two tablespoons of each of the cheeses aside. Spread the polenta on an oiled baking tray, forming a layer about 1 cm thick. Let it cool, then transfer it to the refrigerator for at least an hour (this preparation can also be done the day before, in which case cover it). Briefly dip the sage leaves in a little boiling oil to make them slightly crunchy.

Cut many discs of polenta with a diameter of approximately 56 centimetres, using a pastry cutter. Then place them on a lightly oiled baking tray, overlapping them slightly. Sprinkle with the reserved cheeses, arrange the sage leaves and drizzle with a drizzle of oil. Bake at 180°C for about 15 minutes. If necessary, pass the gnocchi under the grill for a few minutes. Add the chopped walnuts and serve.

BAKED WHOLE WHOLE PASTA WITH PEPPERS AND PECORINO

Difficulty: easy

Time 25 minutes + 40 minutes

ingredients

For 4 people

240 g wholemeal Ditalini

1 kg Mixed peppers

150 g of ricotta

40 g grated Pecorino

100 g of tomato puree, 1 chilli pepper

1 tablespoon Capers

10 basil leaves, salt and pepper

Preparation

Arrange the peppers on the baking tray lined with baking paper. Bake them at 200°C with

grill for 20/25 minutes, lining them so that
they brown evenly. To make peeling easier,
once cooked you can place them in a food bag
and immerse them in water and ice until
completely cooled. Then peel them, peel them
and cut them into small pieces. Finely chop
the previously desalted capers, chilli pepper
and basil. Combine the tomato puree, chopped
herbs and peppers in a bowl. Mix well, then
season with salt and pepper and add the
ricotta and half the grated pecorino. Boil the
pasta in plenty of salted water, drain it al
dente and season it well with the sauce. Then
arrange it in a baking dish (or in 4 individual
moulds). Sprinkle with the remaining grated
pecorino and bake at 220°C for 10 minutes,
plus a few minutes of grilling to obtain an
inviting golden crust.

ANDALUSIAN GAZPACHO

Difficulty: Easy

Time 25 minutes

ingredients

For 4 people

600 g of San Marzano tomatoes

100 g Cucumbers

100 g Red peppers

50 g of Tropea onions

1 clove Garlic

60 g Wholemeal breadcrumbs

100ml extra virgin olive oil

30 g White wine vinegar

Salt, black pepper

10 Basil Leaf, Water

1 teaspoon spicy Tabasco

To serve

Arugula, black pepper

Preparation

Make an incision with a sharp knife on the tip of the tomatoes, on the side opposite the stem, and immerse them in boiling water for a few moments, drain them and cool them in cold water. Remove the skin from the tomatoes, remove the stem and divide them into four parts, removing the seeds, and put them in a blender. Peel the cucumber, cut it into slices and add it to the tomatoes. Peel and slice the onion, peel the pepper, remove the stalk, filaments and seeds if present, peel the garlic and remove the sprout inside. Blend everything with the tomatoes in the blender, add the basil leaves, salt, freshly ground black pepper, oil, vinegar, Tabasco, breadcrumbs and about half a glass of very cold refrigerator water. Blend and add a little water at a time, if necessary, until you obtain a creamy and not too liquid consistency. Store the gazpacho well covered in the refrigerator for at least two hours before consuming it (even during the night it will gain even more flavour). When serving, divide it into 4 bowls or glasses and decorate with a drizzle of oil, a sprinkling of ground black pepper moment and a few fresh rocket leaves, well washed and dried.

CHICKPEA FONTINA AND DRIED TOMATOES CAKE,

Difficulty: Easy

Time 10 minutes + 20 minutes

Ingredients for 4 people

70 g of 00 type soft wheat flour

60 g chickpea flour

60 g dried chickpeas, cooked

60 g of fontina, 2 eggs

60 g Tomatoes in oil

3 tablespoons pumpkin seeds

2 tablespoons Milk

2 teaspoons baking powder

1 bunch marten, 3 tbsp. Oil

Salt, pepper, butter

Breadcrumbs, Arugula

Preparation

Preheat the oven to 190°C. Mix the white and chickpea flour with the eggs, milk and oil for a few minutes, preferably with an electric whisk. Add the chopped marjoram, a pinch of salt and pepper to taste. Drain the tomatoes well in oil and cut them into strips. Also cut the fontina into cubes of about 1 cm on each side. Then add the tomatoes, cheese and chickpeas to the mixture and mix gently with a spatula. Finally add the yeast. Grease well and sprinkle the bottom of a small plum cake mold of approximately 20 x 8 cm with breadcrumbs and pour in the mixture. Sprinkle the pumpkin seeds and bake for 20 minutes. Let the chickpea cake cool before removing it from the mold and cutting it into slices about 1 cm thick. Serve it with a few rocket leaves, a piece of dried tomato and a portion of fontina.

WHOLE WHEAT PENS WITH SPRING ONIONS AND GREEK YOGURT

Difficulty: easy

Time 10 minutes +20 minutes

ingredients

For 4 people

320 g Pennoni rigati

wholemeal pasta

6 spring onions

170 g of Greek yogurt

6 threads of chives

1 teaspoon poppy seeds

extra virgin olive oil, salt

Preparation

Clean the roots and the hardest green parts of the spring onions, then cut them into slices about one centimeter thick. Transfer them to a pan with 3 tablespoons of oil and let them soften over very low heat for 5 minutes. In the meantime, boil the pasta and pour one or two tablespoons of its cooking water into the pan with the spring onions, leaving them on the heat for another 5 minutes or until they become soft but not mushy. Remove them from the heat and mix them in the pan with half the yogurt. Drain the pasta al dente directly into the pan with the sauce, add the remaining yogurt and poppy seeds. Mix and serve immediately, completing the dishes with finely chopped chives and a drizzle of oil.

BULGUR SALAD WITH PEAS, TOMATOES, BASIL

Difficulty: easy

Time 20 minutes + 40 minutes

ingredients

For 4 people

240 g of bulgur, 4 eggs

300 g of fresh shelled peas

300 g of mixed cherry tomatoes

1 spring onion, half a lemon

1 bunch Basil

50ml White wine

extra virgin olive oil

Salt and pepper

Preparation

Boil the bulgur in lightly salted water for 1012 minutes. Drain it, transfer it to a bowl and season it with a drizzle of oil. Mix and leave to cool. Peel and thinly slice the onion. Stew it for about 5 minutes in a saucepan with 2 tablespoons of oil, without letting it brown. Then add the peas and continue for another 5 minutes before blending with the wine. Let it evaporate, put the lid on and cook, adding a little water if necessary and stirring occasionally. Finally, season with salt and pepper and add half the chopped basil leaves. Divide the cherry tomatoes into 24 segments, depending on their size, and add them to the

bulgur together with the peas, now warmed
up. Season everything with a drizzle of oil,
lemon juice and the remaining coarsely
chopped basil. Let its flavor. Boil the eggs for
8 minutes. Remove them from the heat and let
them soak in the pan for another minute.
Then cool them and peel them. Cut the eggs in
half or quarters just before serving, season
them with a pinch of salt and pepper and
arrange them on the bulgur salad.

**CREAM OF BLACK CHICKPEA
WITH BEANS, CARROTS
AND POTATOES**

Difficulty: Easy

Time 20 minutes + 20 minutes

ingredients

For 4 people

250 g of black chickpeas

8 new potatoes

8 carrots

200 g of broad beans

1 clove Garlic

Extra virgin olive oil

Salt and pepper

Preparation

Brush the carrots and potatoes carefully, then wash them without damaging the carrot leaves. Steam the potatoes for 1618 minutes. Instead, sauté the carrots with their leaves in a pan with a spoonful of oil for a few minutes over high heat, then add salt and pour 2 spoons of water. Continue on a gentler heat until the carrots are tender but still crunchy. Combine the chickpeas, the garlic clove and 2 tablespoons of oil in the blender, then blend, adding a little water. You must obtain a thick and homogeneous cream. Check the salt and pepper. Place the cream in cups and immerse 2 carrots in each, leaving the leaves sticking out, and 2 potatoes cut in half, then sprinkle the remaining surface with the previously shelled broad beans. Complete with a drizzle of oil and a little salt.

BUCATINI ARRIVED WITH SAFFRON GREEN BEANS

Difficulty: Easy

Time 20 minutes + 25 minutes

ingredients

For 4 people

300 g Bucatini pasta

300 g of green beans

50 g pine nuts

50 g Sultanas

50 g breadcrumbs

1 clove Garlic

Saffron 10 pistils

4 tablespoons of extra virgin olive oil

10 basil leaves, salt and pepper

For the green bean cream

200 g of green beans, 150 g of tomatoes

1 clove of garlic, salt

Preparation

Check and steam all the green beans for about 12 minutes. Set aside 200 g which you will need for the cream and cut the rest into logs. In a pan, combine the chopped green beans, 2 tablespoons of oil, the pine nuts, the soaked raisins, the chopped basil and the crushed garlic. Cover with the lid and cook for 5 minutes, adding the saffron threads, already toasted and reduced to powder, and the salt halfway through cooking.

Blend the whole green beans, peeled tomatoes, garlic and a pinch of salt until you obtain a smooth cream; add a few tablespoons of water, if necessary, to soften it. Boil the bucatini in plenty of salted water. In the meantime, toast the breadcrumbs in a small pan together with 2 tablespoons of oil and freshly ground pepper. Drain the bucatini in the pan with the saffron sauce, add the green bean cream and mix, diluting with a few tablespoons of the pasta cooking water if necessary. Serve immediately, sprinkling a little toasted breadcrumbs on each plate.

CARROT GNOCCHI

IN FRESH BEANS CREAM

Difficulty: Medium

Time 50 minutes + 30 minutes

ingredients

For 4 people

400 g Yellow-fleshed potatoes

200 g type 00 soft wheat flour

1 egg, 300 g shelled broad beans

100 g of carrots

40 g parmesan, 1 shallot

1 tablespoon tomatoes, pureed

30 g of butter, salt and pepper

Extra virgin olive oil

Preparation

Boil the whole potatoes in their skins for 20 minutes or until tender, then peel them and mash them through a potato masher. Let them cool. Peel the carrots and chop them very finely in the blender (or grate them). Alternatively you can steam them or boil them and blend them until you obtain a cream. Mix the flour, carrots, egg and tomato puree with the warm potatoes and mix well until the dough is no longer sticky. Then let it rest for 1520 minutes. Cut the dough into many loaves with a diameter of 1.5 centimeters and then cut them into many gnocchi a couple of centimeters long. Peel and chop the broad beans (leave some whole for decoration).

Then brown the chopped shallot for a few minutes in a pan with 23 tablespoons of oil, add the chopped broad beans, salt and cook briefly. At this point, add a small glass of water and continue cooking for 5 minutes, then blend everything until it forms a cream. Boil the gnocchi in plenty of salted water, draining them with a slotted spoon (once they come to the surface) directly into a pan where the butter will have melted. Sprinkle them with freshly ground pepper and distribute them on the plates previously covered with the broad bean cream. Complete with whole broad beans and parmesan cheese cut into thin flakes. Serve immediately.

RECIPES
SECOND DISHES

PAN-FISHED SWORDFISH

difficulty: easy

people: 4

preparation: 10 min

cooking: 10 min

ingredients:

4 swordfish steaks

white wine to taste

1 clove of garlic

parsley to taste

thyme to taste

Salt to taste.

pepper to taste.

lemon juice to taste

Preparation

Pan-fried fish is very simple: put a clove of garlic in the pan with some aromatic herbs (parsley and thyme stalks), then drizzle with a drizzle of extra virgin olive oil and heat. At this point insert the fish and brown it on both sides, then pour in the white wine and let it evaporate. Once the alcohol has evaporated, add the chopped parsley, white pepper and salt. Be careful not to overcook the fish: even 5 minutes will be enough if the slice is not too large, but you decide: in general the swordfish must be well cooked, but be careful not to overcook it! If you want an even tastier fish, you can marinate it for about twenty minutes with lemon, oil, peppercorns, parsley stems and salt. Enjoy your meal!

GRILLED SALMON FILLET

difficulty: easy

people: 4

preparation: 20 min

cooking: 7 min

Ingredients:

600 g of salmon in 4 steaks

1 spring onion

2 sprigs of thyme

4 tablespoons of extra virgin olive oil

1 bay leaf

1/2 glass of white wine

Salt to taste. pepper to taste.

Preparation

First of all, let's deal with cleaning the salmon. If you purchased pre-cut slices, you can skip this step. Otherwise, fillet the salmon with a sharp kitchen knife and cut it into rather thick slices, then remove all the bones and wash them under running water. Let the fillets dry. At this point we move on to the marinade. Clean the spring onion by removing the outermost layer and chopping it coarsely. Pour it into an airtight container with the oil, the white wine, the leaves of a sprig of thyme, the bay leaf and a little pepper and finally mix everything well. Take the four slices of salmon with the skin and place them in the marinade, making sure to grease them all over. Close the container and marinate in the refrigerator for 45 minutes, and then for 15 minutes out of the refrigerator. Let's now see the cooking phase of the salmon. Place a grill pan on the heat and bring it to temperature. Take the steaks, drain them from the marinade, which you must set aside, and place them on the hot plate with the skin side facing down. Cook for three minutes (even less if the slices are not very thick). Turn the salmon and cook on the other side for 12 minutes. Remove from the grill and arrange the steaks on serving plates. Season with a pinch of salt, a grind of pepper, a few fresh leaves of the second sprig of thyme and a few drops of oil from the marinade, avoiding collecting the solid ingredients. Enjoy your meal!

MEATBALLS WITH PESTO

difficulty: easy

people: 4

preparation: 15 min

cooking: 15 min

Ingredients:

500 g of minced meat

2 tablespoons of pesto

2 slices of bread

milk to taste, 1 egg

breadcrumbs to taste

flour to taste

1 glass of white wine

3 tablespoons of extra virgin olive oil

Preparation

Soak the bread in milk for about ten minutes. In a bowl, combine the minced meat, the egg, the soaked and squeezed bread and the pesto. Start kneading with your hands in order to obtain a homogeneous mixture, then add as much breadcrumbs as necessary to dry the mixture as soon as possible. It must remain moist and not sticky. Form meatballs the size of a walnut and coat them in flour. As they are ready, place them on a plate. Heat a non-stick pan and grease it with oil then brown the meatballs on all sides. Add the white wine, cover and cook for 15 minutes. Serve them piping hot. Enjoy your meal!

BAKED RABBIT

difficulty: easy

people: 4

preparation: 30 min

cooking: 60 min

Ingredients:

8 rabbit breasts or feet

150 g of vegetable broth

40 ml of dry white wine

aromas to taste

100 g of white onion

1 clove of garlic

pepper and salt to taste

extra virgin olive oil to taste

Preparation

Start by finely chopping the rosemary, the peeled garlic clove and the bay leaf; put them on the heat in a large pan with a little olive oil. Leave to flavor for 23 minutes on a low heat. In the meantime, peel the onion and cut it into thin slices: season it with the thyme, drizzle with a drizzle of oil and transfer everything into the pan, without ever turning off the heat. Add the rabbit pieces and brown on both sides for 34 minutes; season with salt and pepper and deglaze with the white wine. Allow the alcohol to evaporate and add a ladle of broth before lowering the heat and cooking for another 56 minutes. At this point, on the bottom of a baking tray lined with baking paper, distribute the pieces of rabbit that you have browned in the pan. Add the rest of the broth and cook in a preheated oven at 200°C for about 40 minutes.

TYROLEAN GROSTL

difficulty: easy

people: 4

preparation: 15 min

cooking: 30 min

Ingredients:

1 kg of potatoes

100 g of speck

100 g of bacon

4 eggs 1 onion

2 tablespoons of chives

50 g of butter

Salt to taste. pepper to taste.

Preparation

First, peel the potatoes and cut them into 2cm pieces. Boil them in plenty of salted water for 20 minutes. In the meantime, in a large pan, melt the butter and brown the diced speck and bacon together with freshly ground pepper. After they have released some of their fat, add the thinly sliced onion and cook for 15 minutes. Add the boiled potatoes, flavored with the chives and, if necessary, add salt. While all the flavors blend, prepare the fried egg: heat a drizzle of oil in a pan, break the eggs and cook over medium heat for 34 minutes. In fact, the yolk must remain soft. Distribute the potatoes among the plates and complete each one with an egg. serve them and enjoy your meal!

BAKED HAKE FILLETS

difficulty: easy

people: 4

preparation: 15 min

cooking: 15 min

Ingredients:

4 hake fillets

1 lemon

1 tablespoon chopped parsley

2 cloves of garlic

extra virgin olive oil

Salt to taste.

Preparation

First make sure the hake is free of thorns by running a finger over the flesh. Then rinse it under running water and dry it with kitchen paper. Oil a baking tray suitable for oven cooking, large enough to accommodate the fish without overlapping it. Lightly salt the meat, season it with parsley and lemon juice and put two whole cloves of garlic inside. Cook everything at 180°C for 15 minutes or until the fish is tender, then serve piping hot. Enjoy your meal!

OVEN STUFFED POTATOES WITH CHEESE AND HAM

difficulty: easy

people: 4

preparation: 15 min

cooking: 40 min

Ingredients:

4 medium potatoes

200 g of provola

1 bunch of chives

90 g of diced ham

Salt to taste.

pepper to taste.

extra virgin olive oil

Preparation

Since we will keep the potato skin during cooking, wash it well under running water, and also clean it with a toothbrush. Dry them and boil them in plenty of salted water for 30 minutes. Like all tubers, it's best to start with cold water when cooking potatoes. When the potatoes are almost cooked, drain them and let them cool. At this point, cut them all in half and, with a spoon, scoop out the pulp to form a hollow. You can also leave your stuffed potatoes whole, you will have to make a cut and extract the pulp from there. Transfer the mixture extracted from the potatoes into a bowl and mix it with the diced provola and the ham, seasoning with salt and pepper. Add the sliced chives and stuff the potatoes with the mixture. Cook in grill mode for 1015 minutes at 200°C and serve hot, enjoy your meal!

CAVAGE MEATBALLS

difficulty: easy

people: 4

preparation: 15 min

cooking: 30 min

Ingredients:

300 g of potatoes

200 g of cabbage, 1 egg

1 tablespoon parmesan

breadcrumbs to taste, 1/2 shallot

1 small clove of garlic

Salt to taste. pepper to taste.

pre-fry seed oil to taste

Preparation

First, you need to have cooked cabbage. After removing the outermost layer of leaves, cut it into strips and boil it in plenty of salted water for 10 minutes. In the meantime, peel the potatoes and cut them into not too large chunks (the smaller they are, the faster they will cook), and boil them in plenty of salted water for about 15 minutes, until they are tender. Drain the vegetables and mash the potatoes with a fork so as to obtain a not too homogeneous puree and chop the cabbage with a knife. Transfer both into a bowl, add a little salt and pepper and all the other ingredients necessary for the recipe: parmesan, finely chopped shallots together with the garlic, egg and enough breadcrumbs to obtain a moist but not sticky mixture. Form meatballs the size of a walnut (you can flatten them or leave them round) and coat them in breadcrumbs. Fry them in a little oil until golden and crispy and serve hot. Enjoy your meal!

BAKED DUCK

difficulty: easy

people: 4

preparation: 20 min

cooking: 150 min

Ingredients:

1 duck

1 orange

3 sprigs of rosemary

1 teaspoon coarse salt

1 clove of garlic

2 tablespoons of

extra virgin olive oil

Preparation

First, carefully clean the duck, flaming any remaining feathers. Then wash it under running water, both inside and outside, and dry it with kitchen paper. Blend the salt, garlic and a sprig of rosemary in a small food processor and set aside. Stuff the duck with the orange cut into pieces and 2 sprigs of rosemary. Then massage it externally first with the oil and then with the prepared aromatic mixture. Place it in a baking dish with a lid and cook at 230°C for 15 minutes, then lower the temperature to 180°C and continue cooking for 2 hours. Halfway through the two hours, add the peeled potatoes and cut them into 2 cm pieces. Alternatively, new potatoes are also fine. Remove the lid, activate the grill mode and leave it on for 15 minutes to get a nice crust. Serve everything piping hot. Enjoy your meal!

BAKED SALMON GRATIN

difficulty: easy

people: 4

preparation: 10 min

cooking: 20 min

Ingredients:

4 salmon fillets

1 bunch of parsley

1 clove of garlic

40 g of breadcrumbs

2 tablespoons extra virgin olive oil

Salt to taste.

pepper to taste.

Preparation

Place the breadcrumbs, garlic clove, parsley and a pinch of salt and pepper in a small food processor. Blend until you obtain a crumbly mixture with an intense aroma. If you use frozen salmon fillets, you will need to let them thaw completely in the refrigerator before using them. Then place them on a cutting board and, if present, remove the skin with a sharp knife. Rinse them under running water, dry them with kitchen paper and place them on the cutting board. Add a couple of tablespoons of oil to the aromatic mixture and mix. Transfer the fillets onto a baking tray lined with baking paper and then cover them with the mixture, pressing lightly. Cook the fillets at 200°C for 10 minutes, then serve piping hot. Enjoy your meal!

VEGETABLE CRUMBLE

difficulty: easy

people: 4

preparation: 50 min

cooking: 40 min

Ingredients:

4 courgettes

1 white or golden onion

15 cherry tomatoes

100 g of 0 flour

50 g of grated parmesan

50 g of cold butter

extra virgin olive oil to taste

Salt to taste. basil to taste

Preparation

Start by peeling the onion and then cut it into thin strips. Wash the courgettes and cherry tomatoes: cut the courgettes into chunks and the cherry tomatoes into wedges or even just in half. Place a large pan on the heat, heat a drizzle of olive oil, add the vegetables and cook for about ten minutes to cook the vegetables while still leaving them crunchy. Season with salt, turn off the heat and leave to cool. In the meantime, proceed with the preparation of the crumble: place the flour and parmesan cheese in a bowl, add the cold butter cut into cubes, and start kneading with the help of a fork, then work with your hands to obtain a crumbled dough. in refrigerator and leave to rest for a quarter of an hour. Once the resting time has elapsed, line the bottom of a baking tray with baking paper, pour in the vegetables, distribute them well and cover them with the crumble. Cover with aluminum foil and place in a preheated oven at 180°C and cook for 30 minutes. After half an hour, remove the foil and bake for another ten minutes or until desired browning is achieved. Once cooked, remove it from the oven, let it cool slightly and serve it. Enjoy your meal!

TUNA MEATBALLS

difficulty: easy

people: 4

preparation: 20 min

cooking: 30 min

Ingredients:

320 g of tuna in oil

400 g of potatoes

2 organic eggs

fresh parsley to taste

breadcrumbs to taste

extra virgin olive oil to taste

Salt to taste. pepper to taste.

Preparation

To prepare these easy meatballs, start by washing the potatoes well then, without peeling them, boil them in plenty of water. When the potatoes are nice and soft, drain them, peel them and mash them with a potato masher directly in a bowl. Add the tuna drained from the preservation oil and shell it. Then add the chopped parsley, salt, pepper, beaten eggs and enough breadcrumbs to make the mixture workable with your hands. Form meatballs and roll them in breadcrumbs. We recommend frying them in boiling oil for a couple of minutes and drying them well before consuming them. If you prefer cooking in the oven, 15/20 minutes at 180°C should be enough: keep an eye on them and when they are golden brown, take them out of the oven. Enjoy your meal!

BAKED HAKE WITH TOMATOES AND OLIVES

difficulty: easy

people: 4

preparation: 20 min

cooking: 20 min

Ingredients:

800 g of hake fillets

olives to taste

cherry tomatoes to taste

1 clove of garlic

extra virgin olive oil to taste

dried oregano to taste

salt to taste

ground black pepper to taste

Preparation:

recipe for baked hake with cherry tomatoes and olives To prepare the baked hake fillet, start by rinsing the hake fillets under running water, then dry them and transfer them onto four sheets of kitchen foil, season with oil, salt and pepper according to your taste. Separately, wash and cut the cherry tomatoes into wedges. Rinse the olives from their preservation liquid and cut them into slices. Place the cherry tomatoes and olives on the hake fillets and finish with a sprinkling of dried oregano. Close forming small packets and transfer them to a baking tray. Bake in a preheated oven at 180°C and cook for about 20 minutes. Remove from the oven and serve immediately, enjoy your meal!

CHICKEN WITH LEMON

difficulty: easy

people: 4

preparation: 10 min

cooking: 20 min

Ingredients:

500 g of chicken breast

00 flour to taste

extra virgin olive oil to taste

1 lemon, 150 g of water

90 g of white wine, salt to taste.

Preparation

Let's start with cleaning the chicken. If you already have the slices you won't have to do anything, but if you have purchased a whole breast, divide it in half and remove all the fatty parts. Once done, let's see how to cook the chicken breast in a pan: flour all the scallops well and brown them in a hot non-stick pan with a drizzle of extra virgin olive oil. Turn them over after about 3 minutes and make sure they are golden and crispy. When the chicken is ready, remove it and set it aside. In the same pan, pour the wine, water, lemon juice, a pinch of salt and a teaspoon of sifted flour to thicken the sauce. Reduce, stirring occasionally, until the sauce has a thick consistency. Then add the chicken and cook for just two minutes. Serve the scallops with lemon accompanying them with the sauce and vegetables you like best. Enjoy your meal!

BAKED PRAWNS

difficulty: easy

people: 4

preparation: 20 min

cooking: 15 min

Ingredients:

12 shrimp

40 g of lime or lemon juice

60 g of olive oil

parsley to taste

pepper to taste.

Salt to taste.

Preparation

Cut the lime (or lemon if you prefer) in half, squeeze the juice and filter it. Add the oil, washed and chopped parsley, salt and pepper to the lime juice. Blend everything with a mini peeper to obtain the ideal consistency for this recipe. Place the cleaned prawns on a lightly greased or lined baking tray. Season with the emulsion, keeping some aside for a later stage. Now let's see how to cook the prawns: cook in a preheated oven at 250°C for around 810 minutes. Once cooked, remove the prawns from the oven and serve immediately with their cooking juices, adding a little emulsion. Garnish the dish with lemon slices. Enjoy your meal!

VEAL STRIPS WITH ARTICHOKES

difficulty: easy

people: 4

preparation: 10 min

cooking: 15 min

Ingredients:

400 g of veal slices

2 artichokes

1 clove of garlic

1 glass of white wine

3 tablespoons of extra virgin olive oil

1 tablespoon chopped parsley

Salt to taste. pepper to taste.

1/2 lemon

Preparation

First clean the artichokes unless you decide to use frozen ones. Then slice them rather thinly, to make cooking times uniform, and place them in a bowl filled with water and lemon. Cut the meat slices into 2cm wide strips. In a pan, heat the oil with the garlic clove and brown the meat. Then add the artichokes, pour in the white wine and cook over medium heat for 15 minutes, until tender. If necessary, you can add a few tablespoons of water. Almost at the end of cooking, add salt and pepper and season with chopped fresh parsley. To obtain a creamier consistency you can pass the strips of meat in flour before browning them in the pan. In this case it will be necessary to add a little water or broth to cook everything and form the sauce. Serve them on the table, and enjoy your meal!

MEATLOAF WITH ARTICHOKES

difficulty: easy

people: 4

preparation: 20 min

cooking: 45 min

Ingredients:

800 g of minced meat

2 artichokes

3 tablespoons of parmesan

50 g of breadcrumbs

1 organic egg

2 tablespoons of oil

1 clove of garlic

Salt to taste.

pepper to taste.

Preparation

First clean the artichokes by removing the outermost layer of the stem and the tips. With the help of a spoon, also remove the internal beard and then cut them into slices. In a pan, heat the oil with the garlic clove, then add the artichokes and cook over low heat for 15 minutes, adding salt to taste. In the meantime, mix the minced meat, parmesan, egg, a pinch of salt, a pinch of pepper and the breadcrumbs in a bowl.

On a sheet of baking paper, spread a layer of
meat 1 cm thick, giving it a rectangular shape.
Distribute the artichokes in the center and,
using the paper, close. Seal all contact points
well. Use the baking paper to wrap the
meatloaf tightly and close it like a candy,
using two pieces of string. Bake in the oven at
200°C for 30 minutes, remove from the oven
and leave to cool before cutting. Serve on the
table and enjoy your meal!

TURKEY ROLL STUFFED WITH COURGETTES AND HAM

difficulty: easy

people: 4

preparation: 30 min

cooking: 20 min

Ingredients:

3 large slices of turkey breast

100 g of thin ham

2 courgettes, salt to taste.

pepper to taste.

a glass of dry white wine

a glass of broth

extra virgin olive oil to taste

Preparation

To prepare the turkey roll stuffed with courgettes and ham, start by taking the turkey breast slices, placing them on a cutting board, and overlapping them slightly on one side. Arrange the slices of ham and the previously grilled courgettes on top. Roll up the turkey breast and tie the resulting roll with kitchen twine. Place a thick-bottomed saucepan on the heat, heat the oil and brown the roll on both sides. Pour in the white wine and when the liquid has evaporated, add the broth. Cover with the lid and cook for 20 minutes, turning the roll from time to time. Turn off the heat and let cool before removing the string and slicing your roast turkey roll. Enjoy your meal!

TUNA FILLET IN PISTACHIO CRUST

difficulty: easy

people: 4

preparation: 10 min

cooking: 10 min

Ingredients:

800 g of tuna in 4 fillets

4 tablespoons of extra virgin olive oil

200 g of chopped pistachios

Salt to taste.

pepper to taste.

Preparation

Pour the oil, salt and pepper into a bowl and the chopped pistachios into another. Beat the oil well to obtain a well-blended mixture.

Using a pastry brush, brush a skinless and boneless tuna fillet on all sides with the flavored oil. Immediately pass it in the chopped pistachios, turning it so that it is covered on all sides. Repeat with the other fillets. Place a non-stick pan on the heat into which you will have to pour the oil left over from the marinade. If it is finished, however, grease the pan with a spoonful of oil. Heat the oil, then place the fillets on top and cook for 1 to 2 minutes on each side. Depending on the cooking time, the fish will melt more or less when cut. In the end, in fact, the inside must still be red in color, while the external parts must be more cooked. Arrange the fillets on serving plates and serve them on the table, enjoy your meal!

SPINACH OMELETTE WITHOUT EGGS

difficulty: easy

people: 4

preparation: 10 min

cooking: 30 min

Ingredients:

180 g of fresh spinach

120 g of chickpea flour

240 ml of water

1 teaspoon of salt

1/2 teaspoon baking soda

1/2 teaspoon turmeric

extra virgin olive oil

Preparation

First, cook the spinach. They can be used both fresh and frozen, the important thing is that the vegetation water is allowed to evaporate well. Once cooked, transfer them to a cutting board and chop them with a knife. In a bowl, combine the chickpea flour, salt, bicarbonate of soda and a pinch of turmeric to taste to give the characteristic bright yellow colour. Slowly pour in the water until you obtain a batter, mixing with a whisk to avoid lumps. Then add the spinach and mix again. Heat a 22cm diameter non-stick pan and lightly grease it. Then pour in the batter and cook for 810 minutes on each side, turning it with the help of a lid or a plate. Serve hot or at room temperature. Enjoy your meal!

GUINEA-STYLE CACCIATORA WITH OLIVES

difficulty: easy

people: 4

preparation: 15 min

cooking: 90 min

Ingredients:

1 guinea fowl, 1 small onion

2 cloves of garlic

1 sprig of rosemary

2 sage leaves

1 can of tomato pulp

1 glass of dry white wine

4 tablespoons of oil

Salt to taste. pepper to taste

Preparation

First, check that the guinea fowl is very clean and, if necessary, brown the feathers on the stove. Then rinse it under running water and dry it with kitchen paper before cutting it into pieces. Finely chop the onion, garlic, rosemary and sage and brown them in a pan with oil. Add the meat and, after browning it on all sides, add the white wine. When you no longer smell the alcohol rising from the pan's fumes, add the tomato pulp, a pinch of salt and start cooking the meat which will continue for 1 and a half hours. Stir occasionally and, if the sauce dries out too much, adjust the consistency with hot water or broth. Only 10 minutes before the end of cooking, add the green olives. Serve hot. Enjoy your meal!

CUTTLEFISH AND ARTICHOKES

difficulty: easy

people: 4

preparation: 15 min

cooking: 30 min

Ingredients:

800 g of cuttlefish

4 artichokes

1 clove of garlic

2 anchovy fillets

1/2 glass of white wine

3 tablespoons of olive oil

Salt to taste.

pepper to taste

1/2 lemon

1 tablespoon chopped parsley

Preparation

First clean the artichokes: remove the tips, the outer layer of leaves and thin the stem. With the help of a spoon, also remove the internal beard and then proceed with the cut, keeping in mind that the finer they are, the sooner they will cook. Then divide them into four and then in half again, placing them as they are ready in a bowl with water and lemon. In the meantime, heat the oil with the garlic clove and anchovy fillets in a pan, stirring to melt the latter.

Add the cuttlefish (if they are whole cuttlefish, and vice versa cut them into pieces) and cook them for 5 minutes. Add the artichokes, add the white wine and cook with the lid on for 20 minutes or until the cuttlefish are tender. If necessary, add a few tablespoons of water to bring everything to the boil, and don't forget to add salt and pepper at the end. Serve hot, complete with a sprinkling of fresh chopped parsley. Enjoy your meal!

CAULIFLOWER BURGER

difficulty: easy

people: 4

preparation: 15 min

cooking: 30 min

Ingredients:

1 medium cauliflower

1 egg

100 g of breadcrumbs

2 tbsp

of grated parmesan

extra virgin olive oil

Salt to taste.

aromatic herbs to taste (optional)

Preparation

First, remove the cauliflower florets and rinse them under running water. Then bring a pan full of salted water to the boil and cook them for 1015 minutes, until they are tender. Then drain them and transfer them to a bowl. Mash them with a fork and let them cool before proceeding with the preparation. Now all that remains is to add the egg, breadcrumbs, parmesan, and possibly the spices or aromatic herbs. Mix until you obtain a slightly sticky mixture that sticks easily. If not, add more breadcrumbs little by little. Give burgers any size you like. Heat a non-stick pan, lightly grease it and cook the cauliflower burgers for 5 minutes on each side, turning them gently halfway through cooking. Then serve them once they have cooled with a side dish of your choice. Enjoy your meal!

STUFFED ARTICHOKES WITHOUT MEAT

difficulty: easy

people: 4

preparation: 30 min

cooking: 40 min

Ingredients:

8 large artichokes

60 g of breadcrumbs

80 g of grated cheese

extra virgin olive oil to taste

parsley to taste

vegetable broth to taste

Salt and pepper to taste.

1 clove of garlic, 1 lemon

Preparation

First clean the artichokes. In this case, however, you need to remove the hard (or thorny) part, cut the stem and then leave the vegetable whole so that it can be filled. Create a groove in the center by pressing with your fingers and also remove the beard of the artichokes then, while preparing the filling, leave them in a basin of water with lemon juice so that they do not blacken. Now in a bowl prepare the filling for the stuffed artichokes. Mix 2/3 of the breadcrumbs with the cheese. Then finely chop the parsley and the clove of garlic without the stone (if you don't like it you can easily omit the garlic) and add it to the bowl with the oil, salt, pepper and a few drops of lemon to taste. Mix everything together and use it as a filling. Fill the artichokes with the previously prepared mixture, making sure it is sufficiently moist, then place them on a non-stick baking tray or baking dish, complete with the remaining breadcrumbs, a drizzle of oil and bake at 180°C for approximately 2025 minutes. If the second vegetarian dish becomes too dry, sprinkle it with one or two ladles of hot vegetable broth. Enjoy your meal!

CARROT PANCAKES

difficulty: easy,

people: 4

preparation: 30 min

cooking: 5 min

Ingredients:

4 carrots, 2 eggs

2 tablespoons of 0 flour

2 tablespoons grated parmesan

3 tablespoons chopped parsley

1/4 white onion

sunflower seed oil to taste

Salt to taste.

pepper to taste.

Preparation

Clean the carrots, peel them, wash them and chop them with the mixer, then transfer them to a large bowl. Also clean a quarter of the white onion and chop this too in the blender. Add the chopped onion to the carrots and mix with a spoon to mix these ingredients better. Separately, beat the eggs with the flour and the grated Grana Padano. Season with salt and pepper and beat vigorously to avoid the formation of lumps. Add the chopped carrots and parsley. Mix well to combine all the ingredients. Take a pan with a shallow bottom and heat 23 tablespoons of sunflower seed oil on the heat.

Pour the carrot mixture with a spoon creating well-spaced pancakes. Cook in boiling oil for about 34 minutes, then turn the pancakes using a spatula. Continue cooking on the other side to obtain even browning. Transfer the cooked pancakes to a plate covered with paper towels. Continue cooking until the batter runs out. Serve the pancakes piping hot and enjoy your meal!

CHICKEN SKEWERS WITH SOY

difficulty: easy:

people: 4

preparation: 20 min

cooking: 15 min

Ingredients:

600 g of chicken breast

50 ml of soy sauce

10 g of sugar

25 ml of white wine

5 g of 00 flour

Preparation

Start by washing the chicken breast under cold running water. Cut into cubes, removing all the bones and fatty parts of the meat. Form the skewers and proceed to prepare the soy glaze. In a bowl mix the soy sauce with the sugar, wine and sifted flour. Transfer to a saucepan and place on the heat. Cook over medium heat, stirring constantly until the sugar is completely dissolved. Leave to thicken then brush the skewers with the sauce on all sides. Transfer the skewers to a baking tray lined with baking paper and cook in a preheated oven at 200°C for 20 minutes (the last 5 minutes in grill mode), taking care to turn them halfway through cooking so as to obtain uniform cooking. Remove from the oven and serve the chicken skewers. Enjoy your meal!

AUBERGINE AND LENTIL MEATBALLS

difficulty: easy, people: 4

preparation: 20 min

cooking: 35 min

Ingredients:

2 Aubergine

250 g of red lentils

1 carrot.

1 shallot

corn flour to taste,

salt to taste.

extra virgin olive oil to taste

Start by peeling the Aubergine then rinse them under a cold jet, dry them and steam them to soften them. In another saucepan, cook the lentils following the directions on the package. Using the mixer, finely chop the shallot and carrot. Once cooked, blend the lentils and courgettes until you obtain a smooth mixture. Add the chopped carrot and shallot, then season with salt. With wet hands or with the help of a spoon, shape the balls, roll them in corn flour and place them on a baking tray lined with baking paper. Brush the lentil balls without potatoes with a drizzle of oil and cook in a preheated oven at 180°C for 15 minutes. Once cooked, remove from the oven and serve the baked vegan lentil meatballs with a side of vegetables in the salad, enjoy your meal!

CAULIFLOWER CUTLETS

difficulty: easy

people: 4

preparation: 15 min

cooking: 15 min

ingredients:

1 cauliflower

flour to taste

2 eggs

breadcrumbs to taste

Salt to taste.

seed oil for frying to taste

Preparation

First clean the cauliflower by removing the leaves and washing it under running water. Using a sharp knife, cut into slices about a finger thick. Dip them first in the flour, then in the lightly salted beaten eggs and finally in the breadcrumbs. As they are ready, place them on a plate. In a pan, heat a drop of seed oil and fry the breaded cauliflower slices for a total of 15 minutes, turning them occasionally. Once ready, drain them with a slotted spoon and pass them on absorbent paper before serving. To prepare the baked cauliflower cutlets, place them once breaded on a baking tray lined with baking paper. Season them with a drizzle of oil and cook at 180°C for 35 minutes. Served on the table, enjoy your meal!

OMELETTE WITH FAVE BEANS PEAS AND GREEN BEANS

difficulty: easy

people: 4

preparation: 10 min

cooking: 30 min

Ingredients:

200 g of broad beans

200 g of peas

200 g of green beans

5 organic eggs

50 g of grated cheese

1 clove of garlic

vegetable broth to taste

Salt to taste. pepper to taste.

extra virgin olive oil to taste

Preparation

Start by taking the pea pods and carefully taking them all out and then placing them in a bowl. Proceed in the same way with the beans, placing them in a different container. Wash the green beans well, remove the ends and place them in a third bowl. Peel the garlic, take a non-stick pan with a diameter of 22 cm and after adding a drizzle of oil, brown it. When the latter appears golden, remove it and add the peas to the pan, leaving them to cook for 5 minutes. Once the time has passed, add a ladle of vegetable broth and insert the broad beans, leaving them to soak for another 5 minutes. Add another ladle of broth and also add the green beans.

Season everything with salt and pepper and cook for another 10 minutes, letting the broth evaporate without stopping stirring. When the vegetables are cooked, turn off the heat, take a bowl and beat the eggs with salt and pepper, adding the grated cheese. Add the warm vegetables to the egg and cheese mixture and mix until smooth. Add another drizzle of oil to the pan where you cooked the vegetables and pour the mixture into it, covering it with a lid. Cook for about five minutes and when the mixture begins to thicken, turn the omelette and let it cook for another five minutes. The omelette with broad beans, peas and green beans in a pan is finally ready to be enjoyed. Enjoy your meal!

LENTIL BURGER

difficulty: easy

people: 2

preparation: 10 min

cooking: 10 min

Ingredients:

200g canned lentils

1 slice of wholemeal bread

1 onion

1/2 carrot

extra virgin olive oil to taste

Salt to taste. pepper to taste.

1 teaspoon sweet paprika

Preparation

Prepare a sauté with finely chopped carrot and onion. Cook them with olive oil and add the lentils. Leave to flavor with salt and pepper for five minutes, then turn off the heat. In a blender, break up the wholemeal bread soaked in water and blend it together with the lentils. Add the paprika and a drizzle of extra virgin olive oil. Blend again until you obtain a fairly compact mixture. Work the mixture obtained with your hands and give it the classic shape of many round discs. Heat a non-stick pan, grease it with a little oil, and cook your burgers. Brown them for a couple of minutes on each side to form a crust. The lentil burgers are ready! You can accompany them with a salad of raw carrot sheets seasoned with oil, salt, lemon and chilli pepper, or enjoy them inside a sandwich with lettuce, onions and tomatoes. Enjoy your meal!

MEXICAN VEGETARIAN ENCHILADAS WITH BEANS AND VEGETABLES

difficulty: easy

people: 4

preparation: 30 min

cooking: 40 min

Ingredients:

2 cans black beans

1 red pepper

100g canned corn

1 can of peeled tomatoes, 1 onion

1 teaspoon cumin

chili pepper to taste

200g cheddar cheese

1 clove of garlic

extra virgin olive oil tortillas to taste

Preparation

First wash the pepper, remove the core, seeds and internal filaments and cut it into pieces of about half a centimeter on each side. Heat the oil in a saucepan and brown the chopped onion with a knife together with a pinch of salt. Then add the pepper and the well-drained corn and cook for 1015 minutes. Drain the beans and add them to the vegetables, flavoring with cumin and making everything slightly spicy with a little chilli. Let it go for 5 minutes. In the meantime, chop the garlic and brown it with the oil and chilli in a separate pan.

Add the tomatoes and mash them with a fork, cooking everything for about ten minutes. Season with salt and blend everything with an immersion blender. Now that all the ingredients are ready, all that remains is to assemble everything: divide the filling into the tortillas and roll them up. As they are ready, place them in a baking dish with the seal facing downwards. Distribute the previously prepared sauce and complete the grated cheese with a grater with large holes. You can use whatever you like as long as it's sticky. Then bake at 200°C for 20 minutes and serve hot, flavored to taste with fresh chopped parsley. Enjoy your meal!

PEPPER AND ZUCCHINI OMELETTE

difficulty: easy

person: 4

preparation: 15 min

cooking: 30 min

Ingredients:

1 courgette

1 red pepper

6 organic eggs

3 tablespoons of parmesan

2 tablespoons of milk

extra virgin olive oil to taste

sale to taste pepper to taste

Preparation

First, wash the vegetables well. Remove the ends of the courgettes, cut them in half lengthwise and then into chunks. Also clean the pepper from the seeds and internal white filaments and cut it into 4 slices and then cut it into rather thin strips. Heat a generous drizzle of oil in a 24 cm pan and add the vegetables, cooking them over high heat for about ten minutes. Only finally, season them with salt and pepper. Separately, beat the eggs with the salt, parmesan and a spoonful or two of milk. Pour them over the vegetables and close with the lid. Let the omelette cook over medium heat for 10 minutes then, once the surface has thickened slightly, turn it over with the help of a plate or the lid. Continue cooking for a few more minutes and serve. Enjoy your meal!

POTATO AND HAM PIE

difficulty: easy

people: 4

preparation: 10 min

cooking: 30 min

Ingredients:

1 kg of potatoes

2 organic eggs

150 grams of mozzarella

150 g of cooked ham

50 g of grated parmesan

30 g of butter, salt to taste

pepper to taste breadcrumbs to taste

Preparation:

Start by placing the potatoes in boiling water and letting them cook for about 20 minutes. Once the time has passed, drain and peel them, mashing them immediately afterwards with a potato masher. Transfer the puree obtained into a large bowl and season with pepper, salt and parmesan. Mix well, add the eggs and butter without stopping mixing the ingredients. When the mixture appears well blended, take a baking tray lined with baking paper and use half of it to create a first layer. Dice the mozzarella and ham and place them in the pan, covering them with the other half of the potato mixture. Cover everything with breadcrumbs and cook in a preheated oven at 180°C for about 30 minutes. After this time, take the potato flan with cooked ham and cheese out of the oven and serve it while still hot, enjoy your meal!

COD WITH PEARS

difficulty: easy

people: 4

preparation: 15 min

cooking: 40 min

Ingredients:

1 kg of soaked cod

700 g of ripe pears

700 g of potatoes

50 g of pitted green olives

20 g of capers

20 g of raisins

20 g of pine nuts

100 g of tomato puree

parsley to taste chilli pepper to taste

olive oil to taste

Salt to taste. pepper to taste.

Preparation

of cod with pears. Take the cod, cut it into slices of approximately the same size, then place them in a saucepan, cover them with cold water, and place on the heat. Close the lid, reduce the heat and cook for 10 minutes. Drain the fish and let it drain well. Take the potatoes, peel them, wash them and cut them into not too thick slices. Also clean the pears and cut them into cubes. Pour a couple of tablespoons of oil into a saucepan, add the potatoes, pears and season with a little chilli according to your taste. Leave to flavor for a few minutes over medium heat.

Then add the olives cut into slices or chopped, the raisins soaked for a few minutes and well squeezed, the pine nuts, the chopped parsley and the tomato puree. Wet everything with a little water (about half a glass) and cook for about twenty minutes from the boil. After this time, add the cod cut into cubes, and lower the heat, taking care to mix occasionally. Once cooked, sprinkle with pepper and season with salt if necessary. Serve immediately, enjoy your meal!

SEAFOOD SALAD WITH MUSSELS AND CELERY

difficulty: easy

people: 4

preparation: 10 min

cooking: 10 min

Ingredients:

2 kg of mussels

1 large whole celery

extra virgin olive oil to taste

1 untreated lemon

black pepper to taste

Salt to taste.

Preparation

Simple and quick, this recipe will allow you to enjoy a new version of the classic seafood salad, with mussels and celery. The fundamental thing is to ensure that the molluscs are cleaned correctly: then free them from their conservation net and wash them under running water, scratching well, one mussel at a time. Remove damaged mussels. In the meantime, put a very large, capacious pan on the heat and add lots of water. Once you have finished cleaning and preparing all the mussels, throw them into the pan and boil them for about 10 minutes.

minutes, then drain and leave the molluscs to cool, taking care to remove any shells that are still closed. While the mussels are cooling, clean the celery, remove the toughest and most stringy part and cut it into not too thin slices. Separately, squeeze the juice of a whole lemon, washed and possibly untreated, to obtain a small amount of fine zest from the peel, using a grater. Take a large bowl, add the celery, and season with extra virgin olive oil, salt, pepper and lemon juice, then mix well. Take the now hot mussels and add them to the seasoned celery, mix again, and then enrich with the lemon zest. The dish is ready and the addition of lemon zest is perfect, enjoy your meal!

**PORK FILLET
WITH PEACHES**

difficulty: easy

people: 4

preparation: 30 min

cooking: 20 min

Ingredients:

1 pork fillet

6 beautiful ripe peaches

but not too soft

aromatic herbs to taste

1 teaspoon of yogurt

unsweetened white

dried thyme to taste

Salt to taste. pepper to taste.

Preparation

First, wash the peaches well, cut them in half, remove the central stone, then cut the peaches into wedges and then into cubes. Place four peaches cut into wedges in a large baking dish with the thyme, then add the pork fillet cut into medallions, season with oil, salt and pepper, cover with cling film and leave to rest in the refrigerator for an hour. After the meat has rested, pour a drizzle of oil into a pan with low sides, place on the heat and heat. Cook the pork medallions for 45 minutes per side, then add the peach segments from the marinade and cook for a few more minutes. Blend the other two peaches with the yogurt and serve the fillet as desired with the grilled peaches and sauce. Enjoy your meal!

AUBERGINES STUFFED WITH TUNA

difficulty: easy

people: 4

preparation: 30 min

cooking: 10 min

Ingredients:

4 aubergines

500 g of cherry tomatoes

1 clove of garlic

4 tablespoons of olive oil

400 g of canned tuna

2 tablespoons pickled capers

Salt to taste. basil to taste

80 g of grated pecorino

100 g of scamorza

Preparation

of the recipe for aubergines stuffed with tuna Start by carefully washing and drying the vegetables. Remove the upper end, which is tough, and cut them into two equal parts, lengthwise. Using a teaspoon or a sharp knife, remove all the pulp from the aubergines, leaving a 1cm border. Collect the pulp on a pastry board and chop it coarsely with a knife. Heat a non-stick pan, then transfer the vegetable pulp into it. Stir occasionally during cooking. When it begins to brown, add salt and cover with two tablespoons of oil. Once cooked, turn off. Boil the aubergine "shells" in a saucepan full of salted water for 3 minutes over moderate heat. Pour the tuna into a plate and break it into pieces.

Wash and dice the cherry tomatoes, chop the capers and dice the scamorza. Add these ingredients to the tuna, together with the cooked aubergine pulp, and mix. Pour two tablespoons of oil into a pan and add a clove of garlic. Spread the seasoning into the aubergine shells and place them in the pan. Season with salt and sprinkle with grated pecorino, cover with a lid and cook for 5 minutes over low heat. Once cooked, turn off and serve garnished with basil leaves. Enjoy your meal!

PEPPERS STUFFED WITH QUINOA AND VEGETABLES

difficulty: easy

people: 10

preparation: 20 min

cooking: 40 min

Ingredients:

8 round red and yellow peppers

810 tablespoons quinoa (gluten-free)

810 tablespoons of bulgur

16 pitted green olives

2 small peppers, 2 courgettes

extra virgin olive oil salt to taste.

Preparation

peppers stuffed with quinoa and without meat
To prepare vegetarian stuffed peppers, first of
all remember that bulgur contains gluten and
is therefore not suitable for celiacs. If
necessary, you can use only the quinoa or
replace it with another cereal. Cook the cereal
following the directions on the boxes. Cut the
courgettes and chilli pepper into cubes, and
the olives into slices. Drain the cereals and add
the vegetables. Cut the peppers by taking the
cap (keep it aside to close them), and remove
the seeds and the internal white part. Fill
them with oil and salt to your liking and close
them with the vegetable caps.

Place the peppers in the oven in a bowl and cook for approximately 2025 minutes, until wilted. If you use smaller peppers, remember that they obviously cook in less time, although, of course, it all depends on your tastes. Conversely, for larger peppers, cooking times may increase by a few minutes. The choice is yours. Serve your light stuffed peppers piping hot. Enjoy your meal!

CHICKEN WITH PEPPERS

difficulty: easy

people: 4

preparation: 15 min

cooking: 45 min

Ingredients:

1.5kg chicken breast and wings

3 yellow and red peppers

2 tomatoes

2 cloves of garlic

1 glass of white wine

extra virgin olive oil to taste

Salt to taste. pepper to taste,

parsley to taste

1/2 tablespoon of sugar

Preparation

Start by cleaning your yellow and red peppers, removing the stem, seeds and all the internal white parts, then cutting them into strips. Also wash the cherry tomatoes and cut them into chunks. If you have time, remove the skin from the tomatoes, as they will melt from the skin during cooking, which could therefore be unpleasant in the mouth. The procedure is very simple: cut them crosswise, immerse them in boiling water for just 30 seconds and then drain them with a slotted spoon. Let them cool and see that the skin will peel off immediately. Place the chicken in a non-stick pan, after heating a few tablespoons of extra virgin olive oil with two cloves of garlic.

The brown forms the outer crust of the meat. When the temperature is high, add a glass of white wine and add the peppers and cherry tomatoes. Salt and pepper to taste and add half a teaspoon of sugar, to remove the acidity of the tomato. If desired, you can also add aromatic herbs to the cooking. Cook with a lid for at least 45 minutes and, once ready, serve piping hot with fresh parsley. Our chicken is ready. Enjoy your meal!

**STURGEON TURKEY
WITH VEGETABLES**

difficulty: easy, people: 4

preparation: 10 min

cooking: 90 min

Ingredients:

1 kg of turkey

Salt to taste. pepper to taste.

1 stalk of celery 1 carrot

100 g of red beans

1 sprig of sage and rosemary to taste

5 cloves, nutmeg to taste

Preparation

Take the turkey part, wash and clean the meat both inside and out, removing the entrails.

You can ask your butcher to clean the meat. Lay out a thin cloth and kitchen towel and place the meat on top. Complete with aromatic herbs, such as sage, cloves, rosemary, nutmeg and pepper. Clean and wash the vegetables and legumes, such as red beans, carrots and celery, and add these too. Season with salt and cover with a cloth. Fill a pan with water and salt it. Dip the turkey inside and boil on the heat for 1 and a half hours. Once the cooking time has elapsed, transfer everything onto a wire rack. Let the contents cool completely. Next, open the towel and transfer the turkey to a serving platter to cut into portions, also removing the bones. Alternatively, you can also present it to the whole table. Distribute the pulp on plates and accompany it with the vegetables. Enjoy your meal!

CHICKEN ROLLS WITH PESTO

difficulty: easy

people: 4

preparation: 15 min

cooking: 20 min

Ingredients:

8 slices of chicken breast

150 g of Genoese pesto

breadcrumbs to taste

olive oil to taste

flour to taste

Salt to taste.

pepper to taste.

Preparation

some chicken rolls with pesto. Take the chicken slices, place them on a cutting board and crush them lightly with a meat mallet. Spread a generous layer of Genoese pesto on the slices. Roll up the slices and secure them with the help of toothpicks so as to block the edges of the meat. Now put some breadcrumbs and flour on a plate, season with salt and pepper and mix. Dip the chicken rolls in the bread and flour mixture until they are completely covered. Take a baking tray and grease the bottom with a couple of tablespoons of oil. Place the pan on the heat, heat the oil over a low heat then place the rolls on top. Continue cooking until the meat is golden brown. If you want to obtain a light sauce you can add a drop of water during cooking, a real delicacy, enjoy your meal!

**SAVORY PIE WITH
GREEN BEANS AND
COURGETTES**

difficulty: easy

people: 8

preparation: 15 min

cooking: 55 min

Ingredients:

6 organic eggs

120 g of 00 flour

400 g of courgettes

150 g of green beans

300 g of spreadable cheese

80 g of grated parmesan

1 clove of garlic

1 sachet of yeast for savory cakes

extra virgin olive oil to taste

Salt to taste. pepper to taste.

Preparation

of the savory pie with green beans and courgettes recipe. Start by washing and cleaning the green beans and then cutting them into pieces. Also wash the courgettes, cut a few slices to keep aside, and grate the rest by pouring it into a bowl. Take a non-stick pan, grease it with a drizzle of oil and after peeling the garlic, brown it. When the garlic appears golden, add the chopped green beans to the pan and cook for 5 minutes, then leave to cool on a plate without the garlic. Take a large bowl and mix the eggs with the parmesan, flour, yeast and grated courgettes.

Stir to combine all the ingredients and add the cheese and green beans. Season everything with salt and pepper and continue mixing until the mixture appears smooth and homogeneous. Take a 22 cm diameter baking mold, flour it and pour the mixture into it. Lightly flour the courgette slices previously set aside and place them on the mixture. Cook everything in a preheated oven at 180°C and leave for about 45 minutes. Once the time has passed, take the cake out of the oven and let it cool for a few minutes before serving. Enjoy your meal!

SALAD OF MOSCARDINI AND GREEN BEANS

difficulty: easy

people: 4

preparation: 10 min

cooking: 35 min

Ingredients:

800 g of green beans

300 g of octopus

150 g of tuna in oil

1 clove of garlic

extra virgin olive oil to taste

vinegar to taste lemon to taste

chili pepper to taste

Salt to taste. pepper to taste.

Preparation

of the octopus and green bean salad recipe, Start by taking a large pot, pour in some water with a pinch of salt and bring it to the boil. In the meantime, wash and clean the green beans and when the water boils, pour them into the pan and cook for 15 minutes, draining them and setting them aside once ready. In the meantime, wash and clean the octopus, take another pan and cook them in boiling water and lemon juice, again for 15 minutes. Once the time has passed, drain the octopus and cut the larger ones in half. You can leave the little ones whole. Once ready, set them aside. Take another saucepan and pour in a drizzle of vinegar, a little chilli pepper and the peeled but still whole clove of garlic. Bring everything to the boil and let it evaporate for a couple of minutes. Once this is done, turn off the heat and remove the garlic. In a large bowl, drain the tuna and add it to the octopus and green beans. Season everything with a drizzle of oil, freshly flavored vinegar, and salt and pepper to your taste. Mix everything together and place in the fridge until ready to serve. The dish is ready to be enjoyed as soon as it comes out of the refrigerator or left for a few minutes at room temperature. Enjoy your meal!

CHICKEN IN SWEET AND SOUR SAUCE

difficulty: easy

people: 4

preparation: 30 min

cooking: 30 min

Ingredients:

400 g of chicken breast

1 red pepper

3 slices of pineapple

2 tablespoons extra virgin olive oil

1 tablespoon of tomato paste

150 g of sugar

150 g of white wine vinegar

250 g of water 150 g of flour

Salt to taste. oil for frying to taste

Preparation

Sweet and sour chicken recipe. Start by preparing the sweet and sour sauce by pouring 50 ml of water and the sugar into a saucepan and letting it dissolve. Bring to the boil and add the vinegar and tomato paste, stirring until the latter has dissolved. Turn off and keep aside. Cut the chicken breast into pieces of about 1.5 cm on each side. Prepare a batter with water and flour, add salt and dip the chicken pieces a few at a time, draining them of excess batter. Fry them in plenty of seed oil until they are crispy, then drain them with a slotted spoon and pass them on absorbent paper.

Heat the oil in a wok and add the peppers, washed, cleaned and cut into cubes approximately the same size as the chicken. Sauté them for a few minutes then add the pineapple cut into pieces of the same size. Then add the chicken and as soon as the work has heated up, add the sweet and sour sauce, sautéing everything for a few minutes. Serve hot with rice on the side. Enjoy your meal!

THAI CHICKEN BITES CURRY AND COCONUT MILK

difficulty: easy

people: 4

preparation: 15 min

cooking: 25 min

Ingredients:

400 g of chicken breast

1 can coconut milk

flour to taste salt to taste.

1 clove of garlic

1 finger of ginger

2 teaspoons curry

1 bunch of parsley

2 tablespoons of seed oil

Preparation

First prepare the chicken nuggets by cutting them into pieces. Dredge them in the flour, remove the excess and keep them aside. In a saucepan, heat the seed oil and brown the crushed garlic, the peeled and grated ginger and the curry using the appropriate utensil. Then add the chicken and brown it over medium heat for a few minutes. Cover with coconut milk and continue cooking for the next 20 minutes, adding salt to taste. Once cooked, complete with a sprinkling of parsley and serve. Enjoy your meal!

OMELETTE WITH AGRETTI!

difficulty: easy

people: 4

Preparation: 25 min

cooking: 15 min

Ingredients:

5 eggs

200 g of agretti

200 g of fresh ricotta

30 g of grated parmesan

extra virgin olive oil to taste

Salt to taste. pepper to taste.

Preparation

of the agretti omelette recipe Take the agretti and remove all the roots and any damaged stems. Wash the agretti cold running water then boil them in lightly salted boiling water for 34 minutes. Drain the agretti and set them aside for a moment. In the meantime, shell the eggs in a large bowl, beat them with the help of a whisk, then add the ricotta and parmesan. Mix well then add the agretti, pepper and salt. Heat the oil in a non-stick pan and pour the mixture. Cover with a lid for about ten minutes and cook over low heat. When you have to turn the omelette, help yourself with the lid. When the eggs are cooked, turn the omelette and cook for another 5 minutes. Your omelette with agretti and ricotta is ready, enjoy your meal!

SIDE DISH RECIPES

SPINACH AND STRAWBERRY SALAD

Preparation Time: 10 minutes

Cooking Time: N/A

(no-cook recipe)

Dose for 2 People

Ingredients

200 g of fresh spinach

150g strawberries, sliced

30 g of toasted walnuts

50 g crumbled goat's cheese

2 tablespoons balsamic vinegar

2 tablespoons extra virgin olive oil

Salt and Pepper To Taste

Preparation

1. Preparation of the Ingredients: Wash and dry the spinach. Wash the strawberries, remove the stems and cut them into slices. Lightly toast the walnuts in an oil-free pan until fragrant. 2. Assemble the Salad: In a large bowl, add the fresh spinach. Arrange the strawberry slices on the spinach. Sprinkle the toasted walnuts and crumbled goat cheese over the salad. 3. Prepare the Dressing: In a small bowl, mix the balsamic vinegar and olive oil. Add salt and pepper to taste and mix well. 4. Dress the Salad: Pour the dressing over the salad just before serving. Stir gently to evenly distribute the seasoning. 5. Serve: Divide the salad between two plates and serve immediately.

STEAMED BROCCOLI WITH ALMONDS

Preparation Time: 10 minutes

Cooking time: 57 minutes

Dose for 2 People

Ingredients

300g broccoli, cut into florets

30 g toasted flaked almonds

1 tablespoon extra virgin olive oil

Grated zest of 1 lemon

Salt to taste

Pepper as needed

Preparation

1Preparation of the Ingredients: Wash and cut the broccoli into florets. Lightly toast the almonds in an oil-free pan until fragrant and golden. 2. Cooking the Broccoli: Bring a pan of salted water to the boil. Place the broccoli in a steamer basket and place it over the boiling water. Cover with a lid and steam for 57 minutes, until the broccoli is tender but still crunchy. 3. Assemble the Dish: Transfer the cooked broccoli to a large bowl. Drizzle with olive oil and toss gently to coat evenly. 4. Add Seasonings and Almonds: Add the grated lemon zest and mix again. Sprinkle the toasted almonds over the broccoli. 5. Serve: Season with salt and pepper to taste. Divide the broccoli between two plates and serve immediately.

QUINOA WITH GRILLED VEGETABLES

Preparation Time: 15 minutes

Cooking time: 20 minutes

Dose for 2 People

Ingredients

100 g of quinoa

1 red pepper, cut into strips

1 courgette, cut into rounds

1 small aubergine, cut into slices

1 red onion, sliced

2 tablespoons extra virgin olive oil

Juice of 1 lemon

Chopped fresh parsley to taste

Salt to taste Pepper to taste

Preparation

1.Preparing the Quinoa: Rinse the quinoa under cold running water. In a saucepan, add the quinoa and 200 ml of water. Bring to the boil, then reduce the heat and cover with a lid. Cook for about 15 minutes, until the quinoa has absorbed all the water and the grains are tender. Remove from heat and let rest covered for 5 minutes, then fluff with a fork. 2. Preparing the Vegetables: Preheat a grill or grill pan over medium-high heat. In a large bowl, toss the pepper strips, zucchini rounds, eggplant slices, and onion slices with 1 tablespoon olive oil, salt, and pepper. Grill vegetables until tender and have grill marks, about 57 minutes per side. Remove from grill and let cool slightly. 3. Assemble the Dish: In a large bowl, combine the cooked quinoa with the grilled vegetables.

ROASTED ASPARAGUS WITH PARMESAN

Preparation Time: 10 minutes

Cooking time: 15 minutes

Dose for 2 People

Ingredients

300 g of fresh asparagus

2 tablespoons extra virgin olive oil

30 g of grated parmesan

Salt to taste

Pepper as needed

Juice of 1/2 lemon

Preparation

1.Preparation of the Asparagus: Preheat the oven to 200°C. Wash the asparagus and cut the tough ends. 2. Season the Asparagus: Arrange the asparagus on a baking tray. Sprinkle the asparagus with olive oil, salt and pepper. Toss gently to make sure the asparagus is evenly coated with the dressing. 3. Oven Cooking: Roast the asparagus in the preheated oven for 1215 minutes, or until tender and lightly browned. 4. Add the Parmesan: Remove the pan from the oven. Immediately sprinkle the hot asparagus with the grated parmesan so that it melts slightly. 5. Season with Lemon: Sprinkle fresh lemon juice over the asparagus for a touch of tartness. 6. Serve: Arrange the asparagus on a serving plate. Serve immediately.

TOMATO AND CUCUMBER SALAD

Preparation Time: 15 minutes

Cooking Time: N/A

(no-cook recipe)

Dose for 2 People

Ingredients

2 medium tomatoes, diced

1 large cucumber, cut into slices

1/2 red onion, finely sliced

10 black olives, pitted and cut in half

50 g of crumbled feta

1 tablespoon extra virgin olive oil

1 tablespoon red wine vinegar

1/2 teaspoon dried oregano

Salt to taste Pepper to taste

Preparation

1.Preparation of the Ingredients: Wash and cut the tomatoes into cubes. Wash and slice the cucumber. Finely slice the red onion. Pitt the black olives and cut them in half. Crumble the feta. 2. Assemble the Salad: In a large bowl, combine the tomatoes, cucumber, red onion and black olives. 3. Prepare the Dressing: In a small bowl, mix the olive oil, red wine vinegar, oregano, salt and pepper. 4. Dress the Salad: Pour the dressing over the ingredients in the salad bowl. Toss gently to make sure all the vegetables are well seasoned. 5. Add the Feta: Sprinkle the crumbled feta over the salad. 6. Serve: Divide the tomato and cucumber salad between two plates and serve immediately. This tomato and cucumber salad is a fresh and tasty side dish, perfect for accompanying a summer meal or as a light appetizer.

ROASTED CARROTS WITH HONEY AND THYME

Preparation Time: 10 minutes

Cooking time: 25 minutes

Dose for 2 People

Ingredients

300 g of baby carrots

1 tablespoon honey

2 tablespoons extra virgin olive oil

1 tablespoon fresh thyme leaves

Salt to taste

Pepper as needed

Preparation

1. Preparation of the Carrots: Preheat the oven to 200°C. Wash and dry the baby carrots. If the carrots are large, cut them in half lengthwise. 2. Season the Carrots: In a large bowl, toss the carrots with the olive oil, honey, thyme, salt and pepper. Mix well to make sure the carrots are evenly coated. 3. Roast the Carrots: Arrange the carrots in a single layer on a baking sheet. Roast in the preheated oven for 25 minutes, stirring halfway through, until the carrots are tender and lightly caramelized. 4. Serve: Transfer the roasted carrots to a serving platter. Serve immediately. This side dish of roasted carrots with honey and thyme is sweet and aromatic, perfect for accompanying meat or fish dishes, adding a touch of elegance and flavor to your meal.

BAKED CAULIFLOWER WITH TURMERIC AND CUMIN

Preparation Time: 10 minutes

Cooking time: 25 minutes

Dose for 2 People

Ingredients

1 small cauliflower, cut into florets

2 tablespoons extra virgin olive oil

1 teaspoon turmeric powder

1 teaspoon cumin powder

Salt to taste

Pepper as needed

Chopped fresh parsley for garnish

Preparation

1. Preparation of the Cauliflower: Preheat the oven to 200°C. Wash the cauliflower and cut it into florets. 2. Season the Cauliflower: In a large bowl, toss the cauliflower florets with the olive oil, turmeric, cumin, salt and pepper. Mix well to make sure the florets are evenly coated with seasoning. 3. Roast the Cauliflower: Arrange the cauliflower florets in a single layer on a baking sheet. Roast in the preheated oven for 25 minutes, stirring halfway through, until the cauliflower is tender and golden. 4. Garnish and Serve: Transfer the roasted cauliflower to a serving plate. Garnish with chopped fresh parsley. Serve immediately. This side dish of baked cauliflower with turmeric and cumin is flavorful and nutrient-rich, perfect for adding a spicy and colorful touch to your meal.

SPELLED SALAD WITH VEGETABLES

Preparation Time: 15 minutes

Cooking time: 20 minutes

Dose for 2 People

Ingredients

100 g of spelled

150g cherry tomatoes, cut in half

1 medium courgette, diced

1 spring onion, finely sliced

2 tablespoons chopped fresh basil

2 tablespoons balsamic vinegar

2 tablespoons extra virgin olive oil

Salt to taste Pepper to taste

Preparation

1. Preparation of the spelled: Rinse the spelled under cold running water. In a saucepan, bring plenty of salted water to the boil. Add the spelled and cook for about 20 minutes, or until tender but still al dente. Drain the spelled and let it cool. 2. Preparation of Vegetables: Wash and cut the cherry tomatoes in half. Wash and cut the courgette into cubes. Finely slice the spring onion. Chop the fresh basil. 3. Assemble the Salad: In a large bowl, combine the cooled spelled, cherry tomatoes, courgette, spring onion and chopped basil. 4. Prepare the Dressing: In a small bowl, mix the balsamic vinegar and olive oil. Add salt and pepper to taste and mix well. 5. Dressing the Salad: Pour the dressing over the spelled and vegetable salad. Stir gently to ensure all ingredients are well seasoned. 6. Serve: Divide the spelled salad with summer vegetables between two plates and serve immediately.

PEPPERS STUFFED WITH COUS COUS

Preparation Time: 20 minutes

Cooking time: 30 minutes

Dose for 2 People

Ingredients

2 red or yellow peppers, whole

100 g of couscous

150 ml of water

1 tablespoon extra virgin olive oil

50 g dried tomatoes, chopped

2 tablespoons toasted pine nuts

2 tablespoons chopped fresh parsley

2 tablespoons chopped fresh mint

Juice of 1/2 lemon

Salt to taste Pepper to taste

Preparation

1. Preparation of the peppers: Preheat the oven to 200°C. Cut off the tops of the peppers and remove the seeds and internal membranes. Lightly grease the peppers with a little olive oil and place them on a baking tray. 2. Preparation of the Couscous: Bring the water to the boil with a pinch of salt. Pour the couscous into a large bowl, add the boiling water and cover with a plate. Leave to rest for about 5 minutes, then fluff the couscous with a fork. 3. Preparation of the filling: In a pan, heat 1 tablespoon of olive oil and add the chopped dried tomatoes. Lightly toast the pine nuts in a dry pan until golden brown.

Add the dried tomatoes, pine nuts, parsley and mint to the couscous. Season with lemon juice, salt and pepper. Mix well to combine all the ingredients. 4. Fill the Peppers: Fill each pepper with the couscous mix, pressing lightly to get as much filling in as possible. Place the "caps" of the previously cut peppers on each stuffed pepper. 5. Baking in the Oven: Cover the pan with aluminum foil and bake in the preheated oven for 20 minutes. Remove the foil and cook for an additional 10 minutes, until the peppers are tender and lightly browned. 6. Serve: Remove the peppers from the oven and let them rest for a few minutes. Serve immediately.

GRILLED MARINATED COURGETTES

Preparation Time: 15 minutes

(plus 30 minutes of marination)

Cooking time: 10 minutes

Dose for 2 People

Ingredients

2 medium courgettes, cut lengthwise

2 tablespoons extra virgin olive oil

1 tablespoon balsamic vinegar

1 clove garlic, finely chopped

1 teaspoon dried oregano

1 teaspoon dried thyme

Salt to taste Pepper to taste

Chopped fresh parsley for garnish

Preparation

1. Prepare the Marinade: In a large bowl, mix the olive oil, balsamic vinegar, minced garlic, oregano, thyme, salt and pepper. 2. Marinate the Courgettes: Add the courgette slices to the bowl with the marinade. Mix well to make sure all slices are evenly coated. Cover the bowl and leave to marinate in the refrigerator for at least 30 minutes. 3. Prep the Grill: Preheat the grill or grill pan over medium-high heat. 4. Grill the Zucchini: Remove the zucchini slices from the marinade, allowing the excess to drip off. Arrange the courgette slices on the preheated grill. Grill for about 45 minutes per side, until the zucchini is tender and has grill marks. 5. Serve: Transfer the grilled courgettes to a serving platter. Garnish with chopped fresh parsley.

CONCLUSION

Conclusion Thank you for embarking on this journey with "Sonoma Diet 2025". I hope you have found inspiration in the pages of this book to adopt a healthier and more balanced lifestyle. The Sonoma Diet is not just an eating plan, but a way of life that celebrates delicious, nutritious food, wellness and mindfulness. Adopting the Sonoma Diet means embracing the quality and variety of whole foods, enjoying the authentic flavors of Mediterranean cuisine and appreciating every meal as a moment of pleasure and self-care. Whether you're just starting out on your journey or trying to maintain a healthy weight, remember that every small choice can make a big difference in your health and happiness.

Your Feedback Matters If you enjoyed the book and found the Sonoma Diet useful for your lifestyle, I kindly invite you to leave a review. Your feedback is valuable and can help other people discover and benefit from this nutritional approach. Thank you again for your trust and have a safe journey towards a healthier and happier life!

[KLARLOCK]